Nursing Issues

for the **Nineties** *and* **Beyond**

Bonnie Bullough, FNP, PhD, FAAN is a nurse practitioner, a sociologist, and a nurse educator. She contributed to the development of the nurse practitioner role by setting up an Extension Program to prepare Pediatric Nurse Practitioners in 1968 at University of California in Los Angeles, and a Masters Degree program for Family Nurse Practitioners at UCLA in 1972. She was head of the Masters Degree Nurse Practitioner programs at California State University-Long Beach in from 1975 to 1979.

Dr. Bullough worked with members of the California and New York Legislatures to obtain recognition for the nurse practitioner role in state laws and published several articles and a book (*The Law and the Expanding Nursing Role* 1975, 1980) related to the legal struggles of nurse practitioners to make full use of their talents.

She served as Dean of the School of Nursing at SUNY Buffalo from 1980 to 1991, and Professor of Nursing from 1991–1993.

In addition to her publications related to the sociology of the law as it relates to nursing, she also does research and writing related to the history of nursing, community health problems, and human sexuality.

The Bulloughs have established a special collection on the history of nursing at the SUNY Buffalo Health Science library and another on human sexuality at the California State University Northridge library.

Vern L. Bullough, PhD, RN, FAAN is SUNY Distinguished Professor at SUNY College, Buffalo. His is the author, co-author, or editor of some 35 books, fourteen of which are on nursing or health related topics.

Dr. Bullough is senior editor of FREEN *INQUIRY* Magazine, a fellow of the Society for the Scientific Study of Sex, and a columnist for the *JOURNAL OF PROFESSIONAL NURSING*. He has been especially active in the American Association for the History of Nursing and was the first editor of its *BULLETIN*. He has also written for a number of encyclopedias including the *ENCYCLOPEDIA BRITANICA* and the *ENCYCLOPEDIA AMERICANA*.

Nursing Issues

for the Nineties *and* Beyond

Bonnie Bullough, FNP, PhD, FAAN
Vern L. Bullough, PhD, RN, FAAN
Editors

Springer Publishing Company
New York

Springer Publishing Company, Inc.
536 Broadway
New York, NY 10012

94 95 96 97 98 / 5 4 3 2 1

Library of Congress Cataloging-in-Publication Data

Nursing issues for the nineties and beyond / Bonnie Bullough, Vern
   Bullough, editors.
      p.   cm.
   Includes bibliographical references and index.
   ISBN 0-8261-8050-7
   1. Nursing—Practice.   I. Bullough, Bonnie.   II. Bullough, Vern
L.
   [DNLM: 1. Nursing—trends—United States.   WY 16 N974155 1994]
RT82.N866   1994
362.1'73—dc20
DNLM/DLC
for Library of Congress   93-47571
                                                               CIP

Printed in the United States of America

Contents

Contributors

Michael Ackerman, RN, DNS, CCRN
Critical Care Clinical Nurse Specialist
Verterans Administration Hospital
Buffalo, New York

Martha Dewey Bergren, RN, MS
DNS Student
SUNY Buffalo
Buffalo, N.Y.

Bonnie Bullough, FNP, PhD, FAAN
Dean Emeritus
SUNY Buffalo School of Nursing
Buffalo, New York
Northridge, California

Vern Bullough, RN, PhD, FAAN
Distinguished SUNY Professor
Dean Emeritus, Natural and Social
  Sciences
SUNY College
Buffalo, N.Y.
Northridge, California

Nancy Campbell-Heider, RNC, PhD
Assistant Professor
School of Nursing
SUNY Buffalo
Buffalo, N.Y.

Patricia Castiglia, PhD, RNC, PNP
Professor and Dean: College of Nursing
  and Health Sciences
The University of Texas at El Paso
El Paso, Texas

Andrew Feldman, JD
Senior Trial Partner
Damon & Morey
Buffalo, New York

Joy Feldman, RN, MA, JD
General Counsel
Park Associates, Inc.
Buffalo, New York

Linda Janelli, RNC, EdD
Assistant Professor
School of Nursing
SUNY Buffalo
Buffalo, New York

Cynthia Allen Hart, RN, CS, EdD
Consultant, Psychiatric Consultation
  Liaison Nursng
Rochester, New York

Marilyn Hyche Johnson, RN, MS
Clinical Assistant Professor
School of Nursing
SUNY Buffalo
Buffalo, New York

Milene A. Megel, RN, PhD
Executive Secretary
State Board for Nursing
New York State Educational
  Department
Albany, New York

Lisa Monagle, CNM, PhD
Clinical Assistant Professor
Department of Social and Preventive
  Medicine
School of Medicine
SUNY Buffalo
Buffalo, New York

Adele R. Pillitteri, CPNP, PhD
Assistant Professor
School of Nursing
SUNY Buffalo
Buffalo, New York

Mattie L. Rhodes, RN, PhD
Clinical Assistant Professor
School of Nursing
SUNY Buffalo
Buffalo, New York

Yvonne Scherer, RN, EdD
Clinical Assistant Professor
School of Nursing
SUNY Buffalo
Buffalo, New York

Ann Seidl, RN, PhD
Assistant Professor
School of Nursing
SUNY Buffalo
Buffalo, New York

Introduction

Bonnie Bullough and Vern L. Bullough

This is the fifth volume of the Springer series on issues in nursing. The first volume, *Issues in Nursing*, was published in 1966. It was contracted with Bernhard Springer, who had already gained a reputation among nurses for his concern about the issues and problems that they confronted. He was willing to publish such a volume, even though the format was new to nursing, because he could see its value for enhancing discussion. Ursula Springer took over the subsequent volumes, and has remained as loyal to nursing and our concerns as was her husband, Bernhard.

The text for the first three volumes consisted of reprints of articles and portions of books clustered to form a basis for discussion of the problems of the day. Volume IV was a combination of reprints and original articles. This volume is composed entirely of original articles.

The issues facing nurses have changed over time. One of the highlights of Volume I was a discussion about the varied educational systems used for basic nursing education; hospital diploma programs were the most common, with some baccalaureate programs. The community college programs were new and their potential was debated. The question as to whether or not nursing could be considered a profession was also discussed in that first volume. A related issue, although it was not always recognized, was the low salaries and deprived economic condition of nurses.

Volume II, *New Directions for Nurses,* came out in 1971. It reported the beginning of the roles of the nurse practitioner and clinical nurse specialists and analyzed the factors in the health care delivery system, which created the new roles, including the fact that physicians had severely limited their numbers to keep their income high, resulting in a severe shortage of health care providers (Bullough, 1984; Fein, 1967). The nurse

1

practitioners who were described in that volume had very modest roles, restricted to well baby care and physician support services. Within the context of these developments documents were presented tracing the history of the nurse–doctor relationship. Historically, physicians had thought of nurses as uneducated, humble, and willing servants, and some doctors apparently went through significant trauma as their relationships changed to allow even modest levels of autonomy on the part of nurses. It is apparent from the discussions of that volume and the subsequent changes that have occurred that physicians are a major factor in the lives of nurses. However, the reverse is also true; nurses have been a continued source of concern to physicians. The two professions have a significant impact on each other.

Volume III, *Expanding Horizons for Nurses*, dated 1977, reported the positive impact of the women's movement on nursing, and the changes in the Labor Relations Act, which allowed collective bargaining but caused nursing supervisors to leave the American Nurses' Association. These forces were supporting a more independent stance among nurses. The continued growth of nurse practitioners and other advanced practice roles was fostered by changes in state nurse practice acts to accommodate the more autonomous roles. The number of diploma programs had decreased significantly, and the major educational issue of the day was whether or not a baccalaureate degree could be required for all registered nurses or whether nursing as an occupation would become more stratified, with the collegiate educational levels preparing the leadership component of the profession, and the greatly expanded community college sector serving as the major program for registered nurses.

The trends of the 1970s continued into the 1980s with Volume IV, *Nursing Issues and Nursing Strategies for the Eighties*. Those who still hoped all nurses would earn a baccalaureate degree had persisted, and their writing was represented in the volume, but it was clear that the escalating cost of health care delivery, the shortage of registered nurses, and the proven efficacy of associate degree and practical nurses in the clinical settings were strong forces in favor of a stratified pattern for nursing. The hospital diploma nurses, who were the major group when the first volume in this series came out in 1966, had virtually disappeared. Unfortunately, however, the unskilled level of nursing had expanded, and almost half of the nursing work force were nursing aides. This changed the role of many of the nurses with baccalaureate and higher degrees to focus on health care planning and management, so that many of the articles reflected broad issues related to quality control of nursing practice, ethical issues, and ways to foster continued competence.

Volume V, *Nursing Issues for the Nineties and Beyond*, comes out 10 years after the previous volume and almost three decades after the first volume. Nurse historians (including the editors) are now using the early volumes as historical documents. Some of the early issues are no longer problematic. The nursing educational system has improved; the hospital diploma programs have either closed or affiliated with colleges. Nurses no longer seem to worry about whether or not to call themselves professional; it is clear that the advanced levels of nursing are at the professional level, and there are technical and auxiliary levels involved in what has become a complex industry providing nursing care. All levels are important, and a close working relationship between the various levels is crucial.

The changes of the last three decades cause some nurses to complain about the increased pace of their work, their increased responsibilities for administrative tasks, their loss of direct patient contact, and the greater use of auxiliary workers. They worry about unwanted competition from new health care workers, such as physician assistants and new kinds of technicians. Although it is true that these changes have taken place, there are also some new opportunities for nurses. An understanding of these trends can help the profession and the individual nurse to cope with the present and the future.

Current changes are the result of both external and internal forces. The external forces are the stronger ones, and when nursing has hesitated to fill the needs created by those changes, other occupations, such as physician assistants, have moved in to fill the gap. Internal forces within the profession have either facilitated or deterred changes; thus, it is important to understand them. These forces are listed below.

External Forces

1. Development of science and technology has made a wider array of health care procedures possible.
2. The continued restriction by medicine of its numbers has resulted both in high incomes and the almost exclusive deployment of physicians into specialty roles (Office of Technology Assessment, 1986).
3. Changing demographic patterns created patterns of unmet needs, with an aging population, a decreasing birth rate, and increasing immigration of refugees and other Third World peoples.
4. Increased environmental hazards appeared and there was a growth in awareness of these problems.
5. A major pandemic of HIV/AIDS developed, along with epidemics of other sexually transmitted diseases.
6. The health care delivery system failed to keep pace with needs, although there is now some evidence that society may well be ready to deal with some of the inequities in the system.

7. Expanded nurse practice acts were enacted, providing at least limited increase in autonomy and responsibility for practice, although it is clear that further expansion of these acts would make better use of the talents of advanced practice nurses (Safriet, 1992).

Internal

1. An increasing knowledge base and growing sophistication on the part of nurses.
2. A more functional and cost effective stratified system of nursing services, with educational systems that prepare a variety of nursing levels.
3. The development of a significant body of nursing research aimed at developing theory and improving nursing practice.

These forces form the backdrop for the issues discussed in the chapters in this volume. The fact that medicine has restricted its numbers and its scope to focus primarily on high-income medical specialties has resulted in gaps in the health care delivery system that are being filled by the advanced practice nursing specialties. Other forces have supported these developments, including the internal changes that have helped nurses become better educated and more sophisticated about research and theory. The focus of the advanced practice roles has also been shaped by a variety of external forces; the aging population has stimulated needs for geriatric nurse practitioners, while the unmet needs of teenagers for reproductive care and the epidemic of AIDS and other sexually transmitted diseases have been important in stimulating the need for women's health care nurse practitioners and nurse midwives.

The better education of nurses and their increased scope of function makes them responsible for more clinical care. The improved technology used in the treatment of patients has led to significant ethical dilemmas. The environmental crisis and runaway American businesses have created a crisis on the Mexican border; nurses are participating in solutions to this problem. The need for an improved health care delivery system, and an apparent current willingness to extend care to more people, is opening up new opportunities for nurses and new responsibilities for cultural awareness.

The professional issues discussed in the volume are also the result of a changing nursing role. The position of nursing relative to the law has changed, and new responsibilities have created new professional issues. The volume ends with provocative suggestions for rethinking our professional image to make it more congruent with our current responsibilities.

REFERENCES

Bullough, B. (1984). The current phase in the development of nurse Practice Acts. *Saint Louis University Law Journal, 28,* 365–395.

Bullough, B., & Bullough, V. (Eds.) (1966). *Issues in nursing.* New York: Springer Publishing Co.

Bullough, B., & Bullough, V. (Eds.) (1971). *New directions for nurses.* New York: Springer Publishing Co.

Bullough, B., & Bullough, V. (Eds.) (1977). *Expanding horizons for nurses.* New York: Springer Publishing Co.

Bullough, B., Bullough, V., & Soukup, M. C. (Eds.) (1983). *Nursing issues and nursing strategies for the eighties.* New York: Springer Publishing Co.

Fein, R. (1967). *The doctor shortage: An economic diagnosis.* Washington: The Brookings Institute.

Office of Technology Assessment, U.S. Congress, HCS 37 (1986). *Nurse practitioners, physician assistants and certified nurse-midwives: A policy analysis.* Washington, DC: U.S. Government Printing Office.

Safriet, B. J. (1992). Health care dollars and regulatory sense: The role of advanced practice nursing. *Yale Journal on Regulation, 9,* 417–488.

PART I

Professional Issues

Principal Issues

1

Opportunities for Specialty Nursing Practice

Bonnie Bullough and Vern L. Bullough

Although the first job of most new graduates is basic bedside nursing in a hospital, many later seek out specialty roles. The nursing specialties have changed and expanded in the last three decades. They now provide nurses with a wide variety of opportunities for advancement, better salaries, and challenging work roles. One of these specialties, nurse-midwifery, is described in a separate chapter in this book. Examples of other interesting opportunities are described below and a brief history of the development of the nursing specialties is provided.

EARLY NURSING SPECIALTIES

During the first part of the twentieth century, nurse specialists were prepared in apprenticeship programs called "postgraduate courses" and colloquially referred to as "posts." The salary of these specialists was only slightly higher than that of the bedside nurse. Students in the postgraduate courses worked long hours with only occasional lectures. The courses were often conducted by prestigious hospitals, although this was not always the case; some were presented by ordinary hospitals that wanted the free labor of the graduate nurses who came to them for additional clinical experiences. A listing of the postgraduate courses which appeared in the *American Journal of Nursing* in 1931 included offerings by 242 hospitals (Courses offered, 1931). The specialty listed most often was operating room nursing, with 37 courses, followed by obstetrical nursing, with 32 offerings; laboratory nursing, with 22; and nurse anesthesia, with 20 courses listed. Some of the early nursing specialties listed in the *Journal* have now become other occupations, such as laboratory technicians, dieticians, physiotherapists, X-ray technicians, and even operating room technicians although operating room nurses are still struggling to keep a nursing identity.

FROM PUBLIC HEALTH NURSING
TO COMMUNITY HEALTH NURSING

Public health nursing differed from the other early twentieth-century specialties because it emphasized formal education in a collegiate setting rather than experiential learning. In 1910, Lillian Wald set up a cooperative course involving both the Henry Street Settlement and Columbia Teachers College (Goldmark, 1923). When the 5-year baccalaureate nursing programs started in 1916, most of them included an option for public health nursing, so a significant portion of the early public health nursing supervisors and even some of the rank-and-file public health nurses had baccalaureate degrees. After World War II the collegiate educational system was realigned and the baccalaureate degree was conceptualized as a preparatory program for all nurses instead of specialty preparation (Bridgeman, 1953).

Although it had started as one role, public health nursing was split off from visiting nursing early in the 20th century. The separation probably occurred for political reasons. American physicians in that era were staunch in their support of the free enterprise system, and most particularly they defended fee-for-service medical care. They were willing to see home nursing provided by private charitable institutions, but argued that it was inappropriate for the public health departments to provide health services and that public health nurses should not be allowed to provide home nursing care. They also insisted that school nurses refer children to private doctors rather than threatening doctors' incomes by treating ill or injured school children. Health departments and schools were forced to narrow their focus to health teaching and preventive services (Buhler-Wilkerson, 1985).

The Social Security Act of 1965 set in motion forces which have made such a total reliance on the ideology of fee-for-service obsolete. This Act provided federal and state financing for the health care of a significant portion of the population, including the elderly, the disabled, the medically indigent, the totally and partially blind, and children covered by Aid for Families with Dependent Children (AFDC). Later other groups, such as patients needing dialysis services, were added to the coverage. While these programs by no means cover all Americans, more than

40% of health care costs are now provided by federal, state, and local governments. Since another 30% are covered by insurance companies, only a small portion of the system is fee-for-service, so even the most conservative physicians have difficulty claiming it is the only possible model.

Public health nursing has now once again been able to broaden its focus to incorporate home nursing and other curative programs under its umbrella. Moreover, private agencies have also broadened their focus to include more health teaching and preventive services, so the field is no longer split. Reflective of this broader emphasis, the current name for the broader specialty is community health nursing.

Home Health Care

The home health care component of community health nursing has expanded rapidly since 1983, when Medicare reimbursements were changed to a prospective payment system. Since the hospital is now paid the same amount whether the stay of a patient belonging to a given diagnostic related group is long or short, hospitals are motivated to significantly shorten the hospital stay of patients (Mitchell & Dibble, 1988). The shortened hospital stays return many people to the community who are still sick and in need of expert nursing care. As a consequence, the existing visiting nursing services have had to expand, and many new home health care agencies have been started. In 1980 there were 2962 home health care agencies. By 1988 that number had almost doubled to 5653 agencies, and this number is expected to continue to grow (Brault, 1990). Some of these agencies provide generalized preventive and curative services to a wide variety of clients, but there are also many specialized agencies. Some of these services are connected to vendors of technical equipment such as respirators, intravenous and arterial lines, and infusion pumps. Specialized nurses insert intra-arterial lines, administer chemotherapy for cancer patients, and supervise parenteral nutrition. Many of the clients would not survive without this specialized nursing care which is delivered to them at home.

Preparation for these roles varies. Many of the agencies demand registered nurses with a record of several years experience in acute care nursing, while others prefer baccalaureate education because of the broader background it provides, and because there is so much teaching involved in the roles. Family members, friends, and even patients themselves have to be taught how to handle the complex equipment when a nurse is not there, and monitor patients to call for help if it is needed.

The generalized home health agencies use teams of health care workers, including nursing aides with minimal training before employment. This means that a significant component of the role of the registered nurse is the supervision and teaching of other health care workers. Moreover, each of the 6 thousand or more agencies has a chief executive officer (CEO), increasingly, that position is filled by a registered nurse. Sometimes the nurse is not only the manager, but also the owner or organizer of the agency. Although nurses have in the past been reluctant to become entrepreneurs, modern nurses are more willing to accept this role, and are proving themselves to be able owners and organizers of health services (Brent, 1989).

While many home health care nurses are certified as community health nurses, the American Nurses Association will recognize the specialty by offering the first certification examination for home health care nurses in 1993 (American Nurses Credentialing Center, 1992).

Case Managers

Case managers are another recently developed role. Although they work primarily in the community, they are also found in hospital settings. The concept of the case manager was borrowed from social work. Social workers oversee many facets of their clients lives, and they often speak of managing a "caseload." The role of the case manager in nursing follows a similar pattern. Usually the clients need skilled or professional nursing care but do not need it on a 24-hour basis. The case manager assesses the client's needs, plans with the client, provides or secures the needed nursing services, and monitors the client's condition (ANA, 1988).

The Veterans Administration is using case managers in at least 70 of its hospital-based Home Care programs throughout the country. A recent article describing the program at one Veterans Administration hospital in Menlo Park, California, indicates that the case manager serves three groups of patients: the post-acutely ill who need medical and surgical care, the terminally ill, and frail persons who have gone home but are at risk for frequent hospitalization or nursing home placement. The case manager plans with the client and the family, sees that he gets the care he needs, and coordinates services provided by variety of other workers. The care maximizes the capability of the patient to remain at home, delaying nursing home placement and avoiding unnecessary hospitalizations. Some of the Veterans Administration programs use nurse practitioners as case managers, while others use clinical nurse specialists (Schroer, 1991).

Case managers have also been useful in the management of chronically ill clients with physical disabilities (Christianson, Applebaum, Careagno, & Phillips, 1988). Patients with mental health problems can often stay out of the hospital if they take their medicine regularly and are able to call on the nurse for support during stressful periods. The nurse visits or calls the client to check that the medication is being taken, helps the client with problemsolving, and is available when needed. Nurse case managers have improved the lives of these clients remarkably. Moreover, they are cost-effective because they prevent unnecessary hospitalization (Franklin, Slovitz, Mason, Clements, & Miller, 1987).

CRITICAL CARE NURSES

Improvements in health care technology provided another impetus for the development of the specialty level of nursing. Most notable were the specialized coronary and other intensive care units in hospitals (Dracup & Marsden, 1990). Most of the specialists who staffed these units are prepared in short-term certificate programs supplemented by on-the-job training. Critical care nurses are the largest group of specialty nurses (Hartshorn, 1988). The membership of the American Association of Critical Care Nurses is more than 68 thousand, with 25 thousand certified as Critical Care Registered Nurses (CCRN). The first master's degree program in critical care nursing opened in Long Beach in 1977, and there are now 20 masters programs. Both the certificate and master's degree programs will probably continue, with the master's and doctoral prepared nurses serving as clinical specialists in the field and teaching critical care nursing.

OTHER CLINICAL NURSE SPECIALISTS

Specialty education became the focus of graduate education after 1965 when the nurse training act (Title 8 of the Public Health Service Act) was implemented (Kalisch, 1982). This legislation was aimed at strengthening nursing education by furnishing funds to enable collegiate schools of nursing to develop master's degree programs. The nurse educators decided that the specialists they were developing, called clinical nurse specialists (CNS), would be bedside nurses who would provide social and psychological support, teach patients and their families how to handle problems related to illness, and serve as consultants and role models to other members of the health care team. The CNS role was also perceived as a way to keep talented nurses in direct care positions (Holt, 1987).

Some clinical nurse specialists focus on a broad field, such as obstetrics or psychiatric or adult nursing, while others narrow their area of expertise to fields such as cardio pulmonary or oncology nursing. Since the primary focus for a CNS is on the non medical aspects of care, these specialists think of themselves as parallel to doctors, rather than overlapping roles with them. When this role first developed the job market was slow, and many CNSs were forced to take supervisory or teaching positions rather than work as clinicians. Eventually the system became educated to the worth of the CNS and the job market has improved, although it is still true that more CNSs than nurse practitioners work outside of their field in nonclinical positions such as teaching and supervision (Elder & Bullough, 1990).

The American Nurses Association certifies four groups of clinical specialists who hold master's degrees: medical surgical, child and adolescent, adult psychiatric and mental health, and child adolescent and psychiatric mental health. However, the ANA also certifies some other clinicians at the baccalaureate or "generalist" level, calling them "certified" registered nurses (RN-C). Those specialties include gerontological, college health, maternal and child health, medical surgical, high-risk perinatal, and community health nursing. ANA has now certified about 90 thousand nurses, with about two thirds of them being either certified registered nurses or clinical nurse specialists; the other ANA-certified nurses are administrators and nurse practitioners (American Nurses Credentialing Center, 1992).

NURSE PRACTITIONERS

Although nurses practitioners (NPs) developed at the same time as clinical specialists, the early training programs started outside the mainstream of nursing education. The major impetus for their development was a shortage of physicians which became acute in the 1960s and 1970s (Fein, 1967). The first formal educational program for NPs was established as a certificate program at the University of Colorado. It prepared Pediatric Nurse Associates (Practitioners) in a 4-month program which included both a didactic component and a clinical preceptorship. NPs work collaboratively with physicians to care for patients with minor acute and stable chronic illnesses. They provide anticipatory guidance to mothers concerning child development, and teach people of all ages how to prevent illness and manage chronic health problems. At the time this role was developed in the 1960s and 1970s, the new knowledge base was drawn primarily from medicine, but the NP positions gave nurses more access to patients and more opportunities to use their existing nursing knowledge.

While nurse educators of that era tended to be enthusiastic about the development of the CNS role, many of them questioned the validity of the NP role. This lack of acceptance was a barrier to the early institutionalization of NP education into the mainstream of nursing education. Gradually, however, the hostility and fears lessened, federal grants provided positive motivation, and the programs were accepted into the nursing schools at the masters degree level (Geolot, 1987; Sultz, Henry, Kinyon, Buck, & Bullough, 1983). By 1980 the master's programs were in the majority, and in 1990 there were 135 master's degree and 40 certificate programs.

Five major nurse practitioner specialties have now emerged: pediatric, adult, geriatric, women's, and family health care. The American Nurses Association, which certifies all of the NP specialties except women's health care, started requiring a master's degree for certification in 1993. Women's health care specialists, (or obstetrical gynecological NPs) are certified by the Women's Health, Obstetric and Neonatal Nurses (AWHONN), which does not require a master's degree. Another separate organization, the National Association of Pediatric Nurse Associates and Practitioners (NAPNAP), the largest certifying body for pediatric nurses, requires the master's degree.

Because NPs overlap with physicians, they also faced resistance from the medical establishment. However, NPs have been shown to deliver high-quality, cost-effective services in a wide variety of studies. These studies were reviewed and favorably evaluated by the Office of Technology Assessment (Feldman, Ventura, & Crosby, 1987; OTA, 1986). More recently, Barbara J. Safriet carefully reviewed the history and scope of nurse practitioner and nurse midwifery practice, concluding that more effective use of these advanced practice nurses could result in significant savings for the health care delivery system (1992).

State Licensure

As the role of the nurse practitioner developed in the mid-1960s it became clear that it would not be legal in most of the states, since most state nurse practice acts included a prohibition against nurses diagnosing and treating patients. Nurse practitioners therefore sought changes in the practice acts that would allow them to practice. At first the deletion of the prohibitions against diagnosis and treatment seemed sufficient, but as the nurse practitioner role developed it became apparent that positive statements in the practice acts were needed to allow NPs to order laboratory tests and prescribe drugs. By 1975 states had started certifying or accepting the national certification of nurse practitioners, nurse midwives, and nurse anesthetists (Bullough, 1980; Bullough, 1984). As indicated in Chapter 3, some states have now moved to full licensure for these three types of specialties. It is anticipated that this trend will continue as the role of the nurse practitioner continues to expand and evolve (Mezey & McGivern, 1993).

SHOULD THE ROLES OF THE NURSE PRACTITIONER AND CLINICAL NURSE SPECIALIST BE MERGED?

The American Nurses Association has proposed that the roles of the master's level nurse practitioner and clinical nurse specialist be merged so all of the master's-level specialists could be called "Advanced Practice Nurses." Research done by Ruth Elder and Bonnie Bullough (1990) indicated that the actual work roles of the two groups of specialists are similar in many ways. Nurse practitioners actually engage in as much patient teaching and support as do clinical nurse specialists, although NPs are less likely to be in administration or academic nursing education. Clinical nurse specialists are less likely to prescribe drugs or order laboratory tests, but additional education could prepare them for these aspects of the role. Merger of these roles would make this group of specialists more politically viable in speaking out on reimbursement issues in Washington and at the state government level.

This proposed merger is however, not without controversy. The title "nurse practitioner" is well-known to the public and it is the specialty that is most likely to be licensed by the states. In addition nurse practitioners believe that the clinical nurse specialists are poorly prepared for patient assessment and management, so the majority of the nurse practitioners are unwilling to participate in the merger. Many clinical nurse specialists, on the other hand, look down on nurse practitioners because of their close association with physicians and because many of them have been prepared in certificate rather than master's programs.

NURSE ANESTHESIA

One of the oldest and most well-developed specialties is nurse anesthesia. Nurses had started administering anesthesia as early as 1889, particularly in Catholic hospitals. Using an apprenticeship format, the first formal course for nurse anesthetists was offered in Portland, Oregon, in 1909. At that time, physician anesthesiologists had no formal training;

interns or colleagues of the surgeon were often pressed into service, so the trained nurse anesthetists were usually the most well prepared people in the field (Thatcher, 1953).

As the specialty of medical anesthesiology developed a turf battle developed, and law suits were brought by medical societies against nurse anesthetists and the hospitals or doctors who employed them. The nurse anesthetists won these cases and the medical societies were unable to get rid of them (Gunn, 1984).

The American Association of Nurse Anesthetists established a certification program in 1945, and an accreditation program to monitor the quality of anesthesia programs followed in 1952. Today there are 22 thousand Certified Registered Nurse Anesthetists (CRNA). Approximately half of the anesthesia given in American operating rooms is administered by CRNAs working with anesthesiologists; CRNAs working alone administer 20%, and physician anesthesiologists the other 30% (American Association of Nurse Anesthetists, 1990). Although most nurse anesthetists were trained in certificate programs, the future trend will emphasize collegiate education. The American Association of Nurse Anesthetists mandated a baccalaureate degree for certification in 1987; a master's degree in nurse anesthesia will be required for certification in 1998 (Gunn, 1984).

NURSING SPECIALTIES

In addition to these master's degree-level specialties, there are many nursing specialties which require shorter, certificate programs; some can still be learned on the job. The larger nursing specialties are listed in Table 1.1. In addition to the ones described above, there are at least 20 other groups that are large enough to have established an organization or association. In general these specialties pay significantly higher salaries than basic nursing, with the licensed specialties and most particularly nurse anesthesia paying the most.

TOPICS FOR DISCUSSION

1. What types of experiences and education would be best for a nurse who wants to work in home health care?
2. Should the roles of the nurse practitioner and clinical specialist be merged?
3. Describe the work role of a nurse you have seen working in a specialty.
4. What are the advantages and disadvantages of the role of the nurse anesthetist?

TABLE 1.1 The Major Nursing Specialties and Their Organizations

Specialty and organization	Members
Clinical nurse specialist (CNS)	
American Nurses' Association	30,000
Medical-surgical CNS	
Psychiatry/Mental health CNS	
Child and Adolescent psychiatric CNS	
High risk perinatal CNS	
Maternal and child CNS	
Community health nurses	
American Public Health Association	2,400
Critical care nurses	
American Association of Critical Care Nurses	72,800
Cardiac	
Surgical	
Medical	
Trauma	
Neonatal/pediatrics	
Diabetes educators	
American Association of Diabetes Educators	7,600
Emergency nurses	
Emergency Nurses Association	22,200
Flight nurses	
National Flight Nurses Association	1,700
Gastroenterology Nurses	
Society of Gastroenterology Nurses and Associates	6,200
Infection control nurses	
American Association for Practitioners in Infection Control	9,000
Intravenous nurses	
Intravenous Nurses Association	8,400
Nephrology nurses	
American Nephrology Nurses	7,300
Neuroscience nurses	
American Association of Neuroscience Nurses	3,700
Nurse anesthetists	
American Association of Nurse Anesthetists	25,800
Nurse midwives	
American College of Nurse-Midwifery	4,300
Nurse Practitioners	
National Alliance of Nurse Practitioners	30,000
American Academy of Ambulatory Care Nursing	1,000
Occupational Health nurses	
American Association of Occupational Health Nurses	12,500
Oncology nurses	
Oncology Nurses Society	23,000
Operating room nurses	
Association of Operating Room Nurses	48,500
Orthopedic nurses	
National Association of Orthopedic Nurses	9,500

(*continued*)

TABLE 1.1 (*continued*)

Specialty and organization	Member
Ophthalmic registered nurses	
American Society of Ophthalmic Registered Nurses	1,700
Plastic and Reconstructive Surgery nurses	
American Society of Plastic and Reconstructive	
Surgical Nurses	1,300
Pediatric Nurse Practitioners	
National Association of Pediatric Nurse Associates	
and Practitioners	4,100
Pediatric Oncology nurses	
Association of Pediatric Oncology Nurses	1,500
Post Anesthesia nurses	
American Society of Post Anesthesia Nurses	9,300
Psychiatric nurses: (Clinical Nurse Specialists)	
American Psychiatric Nurses' Association	2,300
Rehabilitation nurses	
Association of Rehabilitation Nurses	8,600
School nurses	
National Association of School Nurses	8,079
Spinal Cord Injury nurses	
American Association of Spinal Cord Injury Nurses	1,500
Urological nurses	
American Urological Association	2,400
Womens Health Care Nurses	
Association of Women's Health, Obstetric and	
Neonatal Nurses	27,500
Womens Health Care Nurse Practitioners	
National Association of Nurse Practitioners in	
Reproductive Health	1,300

REFERENCES

American Association of Nurse Anesthetists. (1990). Executive Summary. In *The report of the National Commission on Nurse Anesthesia Education* (p. 1). Park Ridge, IL: Author.

American Nurses' Association. (1988). *Nursing case management.* Kansas City, MO: Author.

American Nurses Credentialing Center. (1992). *Credentialing News,* 1, 1.

Brault, G. L. (1990). Home health care nursing: The changing picture. In B. Bullough & V. Bullough (Eds.), *Nursing in the community* (pp. 274–295).

Brent, N. J. (1989). Home health care nurses as Entrepreneurs: Exploring the possibility of establishing one's own home care agency. *Home Health Care Nurse, 7,* 6–7.

Bridgeman, M. (1953). *Collegiate education for nursing.* New York: Russell Sage Foundation.

Buhler-Wilkerson, K. (1985). Public health nursing in sickness and in health. *American Journal of Nursing, 85,* 1155.

Bullough, B. (1980) *The law and the expanding nursing role,* (2d ed.) New York: Appleton-Century-Crofts.

Bullough, B. (1984). The current phase in the development of Nurse Practice Acts. *The St. Louis University Law Journal, 28,* 365–395.

Bullough, B. (1990). Advanced specialty practice: Its development and legal authorization. In N. Chaska (Ed.), *The nursing profession: Turning points* (pp. 375–384). St Louis: Mosby, pp. 375–384.

Christianson, J. B., Applebaum, R., Carcagno, G., and Phillips, B. (1988). Organizing and delivering case management services: Lessons from the National Long Term Care Channeling Demonstration. *Home Health Care Services Quarterly, 9,* 7–27.

The Committee for the Study of Nursing Education, (1923) J. Goldmark, Director *Nursing and Nursing Education in United States,* New York: Macmillan.

Courses Offered for Graduate Nurses. (1931). *American Journal of Nursing, 31,* 612–615.

Dracup, K., & Marsden, C. (1990). Critical care nursing: Perspectives and challenges. In N. Chaska (Ed.), *The nursing profession: Turning points* (pp. 304–311). St. Louis, MO: Mosby.

Elder, R. G., & Bullough, B. (1990). Nurse practitioners and clinical specialists: Are the roles merging? *Clinical Nurse Specialist, 4,* 78–84.

Ethridge, P., & Lamb, G. S. (1989). Professional nursing case management improves quality, access and costs. *Nurse Management, 20,* 30–35.

Fein, R. (1967). *The doctor shortage: An economic analysis.* Washington, DC: Brookings Institution.

Feldman, M. J., Ventura, M. R., & Crosby, F. (1987). Studies of N.P. effectiveness. *Nursing Research, 36,* 303–308.

Franklin, J. L., Slovitz, B., Mason, M., Clemons, J. R., & Miller, G. (1987). An evaluation of case management. *American Journal of Public Health, 77,* 674–678.

Geolot, D. (1987). Nurse practitioner education: Observations from a national perspective. *Nursing Outlook, 35,* 132–135.

Gunn, I. (1984). Professional territoriality and the anesthesia experience. In B. Bullough, V. Bullough, & M. C. Soucup (Eds.), *Nursing issues and nursing strategies for the eighties* (pp. 155–168). New York: Springer Publishing Co.

Hartshorn, J. (1988). The President's message: It's up to you. *Focus on Critical Care, 15,* 67–69.

Holt, F. M. (1987). Developmental stages of the CNS Role. *Clinical Nurse Specialist, 1,* 116–118.

Kalisch, B. J., & Kalisch, P. A. (1982). *Politics of nursing.* Philadelphia: Lippincott.

Mezey, M. D., & McGovern, D. O. (1993). *Nurses, nurse practitioners: Evolution to advanced practice.* New York: Springer Publishing Co.

Mitchell, M., & Debble S. (1988). Acute Care Nursing: impact of DRGs. In *Impact of DRGs on Nursing.* Washington D.C. US Govt Printing Office. Department HHS. Division of Nursing HRSA 87-338.

Office of Technology Assessment. (1986). *Nurse practitioners, physician assistants and certified nurse-midwives: A policy analysis.* Washington, DC: U.S. Government Printing Office.

Safriet, B. J. (1992). Health care dollars and regulatory sense: The role of advanced practice nursing. *Yale Journal on Regulation, 9,* 418–488.

Schroer, K. (1991). Case management: Clinical nurse specialist, converging roles. *Clinical nurse specialist, 5,* 189–194.

Sultz, H. A., Henry, O. M., & Kinyon, J., Buck, G. M., & Bullough, B. (1983). Nurse practitioners: A decade of change, program highlights: I, *Nursing Outlook, 31,* 138–141.

Thatcher, V. S. (1953). *A history of anesthesia: With emphasis on the nurse specialist.* Philadelphia: Lippincott.

2

Nursing Organizations

Bonnie Bullough and Vern L. Bullough

In 1944 the leadership of the three major national organizations of nurses, the American Nurses Association (ANA), the National League for Nursing Education (NLNE), and the National Organization of Public Health Nurses (NOPHN), met to talk about a merger. Leaders of the profession as well as these three organizations argued that seven national organizations were too many. They overlapped with each other and fragmented the power of the profession in the political arena. The slogan "one strong voice" was often mentioned in the literature of the time, and ANA subsequently used it as a title for a history of the organization.

Each of the three major groups carried out a careful study of their structure and functions to see if a merger would be possible. The smaller nursing organizations were also asked to join, and in 1952 the ANA absorbed the National Association of Colored Graduate Nurses (NACGN), pledging to speak out against discrimination in both the association and the profession, so that the NACGN would not be needed. The National League for Nursing took over the responsibilities of three former groups, the Association of Collegiate Schools of Nursing (ACSN), the NOPHN and the NLNE. Only two small organizations remained outside the merger: the American Association of Industrial Nurses (AAIN), and the American Association of Nurse Anesthetists (AACN) (Bullough & Bullough, 1978).

As we look back on that effort after 40 years have passed, the first observation which can be made is that there are now approximately 45 national nursing organizations. The number is an estimate; Americans tend to carry out many functions through voluntary organizations, and new organizations are being formed all the time. However, it seems reasonable to conclude that the 1952 effort to merge and restrict the number of nursing organizations did not succeed. Why was it unsuccessful, and should we again be trying to merge and eliminate organizations?

The numbers and diversity of nurses make such a plan difficult. The nursing work force is the largest occupational group in the health care industry including 1.7 million active registered nurses and 887,000 licensed practical nurses. Moreover, it is a highly stratified occupation. Nurses are prepared in a variety of educational programs lasting from 1 year for practical nurse programs to 8 or more years for doctoral preparation. Nurses are even licensed by the states at three different levels: practical nursing, registered nursing, and the developing specialty level of licensure.

Efforts were made in the 1970s and 1980s to eliminate some of these levels of education and licensure by lobbying state legislatures to change the nurse practice acts to make the baccalaureate degree the requirement for basic licensure. Such a plan proved politically unfeasible, because it did not appear to be cost-effective. Providers argued that many nursing roles do not require baccalaureate preparation and it would increase the cost of health care. The health care delivery system has in fact become even more stratified, and in addition, nursing has become more diversified as the specialty level of nursing has developed.

It now seems apparent that one or two organizations cannot cover all of the needs of so many nurses. These needs include representation of the workers with employers (collective bargaining); political representation, at both the state and national levels; continuing education; certification of specialists; accreditation of educational programs; quality control of practice; public relations; communication; and mutual support. Some of these organizational functions, such as the need for communication and mutual support, are in fact easier to accomplish in smaller groups in which members can have face-to-face interaction with colleagues. The many smaller organizations also allow more people to fill leadership positions. Consequently, the proliferation of organizations was probably inevitable.

The major disadvantage of the proliferation of organizations is the potential loss of political power, since no one group can speak for all of nursing. However, this situation may not be as bad as it seems. Several coordinating groups have grown up to communicate across organizational lines and coordinate coalitions of organizations around political agendas. Particularly important in the political arena is the Tri-Council of Nursing, which started in the 1970s with Washington meetings of representatives of the ANA, NLN, and the American Association of Colleges of Nursing (AACN). In the 1980s the American Organization of Nurse Executives joined the caucus. This group usually sets the major Washington agenda for the profession. The National Alliance of Nurse Practitioners brings together twelve nurse practitioner organizations, and the National Federation of Specialty Organizations brings together approximately 38 specialty groups.

THE SPECIALTY NURSING ORGANIZATIONS

The specialty groups may in fact be one of the reasons why so many nursing organizations are needed. Each specialty group represents nurses with differing needs for continuing education, communication, mutual support, and political activities. The larger or stronger clinical groups also provide quality control through certification and accreditation of programs. The development of advanced specialties, most of which now require master's level preparation, is described in the first chapter of this book.

As indicated above, representatives of approximately 34 of the specialties meet together as the National Federation of Specialty Nursing Organizations. The group was first called together in 1972 by the ANA, with subsequent meetings hosted by other organizations. The affiliation is a loose one and the primary function is communication, although occasionally there will be an issue on which there is a consensus. Member organizations are made up of registered nurses. If the parent body is non-nursing (as is the case with the American Public Health Association) the nursing contingent must have a special section to be included in NFSNO.

AMERICAN NURSES ASSOCIATION

There are, however, many functions which only a broad-based, multi-purpose organization can fill, and for that reason the American Nurses Association is the major organization of the profession. The American Nurses Association was established in 1896 by members of the Society of Superintendents of Training Schools for Nurses of the United States and Canada who realized that a rank-and-file nursing organization was needed. The 1896 meeting brought together members of the Bellevue and Illinois Training Schools, with other schools providing members soon after. The first name taken by the group was the Nurses' Associated Alumnae of United States and Canada, but the Canadians soon dropped out to form their own group, and the group changed its name to the ANA in 1912.

Early efforts of the members of the Associated Alumnae and then the ANA were focused on the campaign for state registration for nurses. Although the first licensure laws were passed in 1903, it was not until 1923 that enabling legislation for registered nurses was passed in all of the states. To facilitate the lobbying effort, constituent state organizations were set up (Bullough, 1980).

The official journal of the association, *The American Journal of Nursing*, was established in 1900 and it continues to be published with a broad focus on the concerns of the profession.

Since most nurses of this period worked as independent contractors in private duty, they needed a mechanism to secure placements, so many state and local associations affiliates of ANA established registries to assist nurses in securing employment. Hospitals were staffed primarily by students until well into the 1930s, at which time staff nursing emerged as the major job market. As the nursing work force changed to reflect the position of hospital nurses, it became clear that support for this group was needed; but the effort to improve the economic conditions of staff nurses faced many barriers, including a reluctance on the part of many ANA members to be concerned about salaries.

Efforts toward collective bargaining started with members of the California Nurses Association during World War II, but these had to be abandoned when ANA ruled the organization would not allow collective bargaining. However, the issue was debated by the membership, and in 1946 the house of delegates adopted an economic program that included collective bargaining, a 40-hour week, and increased participation of nurses in planning for nursing services, but also stated that under no circumstance would nurses go on strike. Unfortunately, the 1947 Taft-Hartley Labor Management Relations Act exempted nonprofit hospitals from an obligation to bargain with their employees, and given the nurses' "no strike" pledge, the hospitals realized they did not need to participate in any collective bargaining with nurses. The right to organize and to strike was finally recognized in 1974 when the National Labor Relations Act was extended to nonprofit health care institutions.

The actual work of collective bargaining is now carried out by the state nursing associations, and collective bargaining has become a major function of the association. This has resulted in a change in the configuration of the ANA membership after an exodus of nurse administrators who were a dominant voice in the early years of the association. They have been replaced by rank-and-file members who participate in state collective bargaining efforts, with nurse educators often functioning in leadership roles (Bullough & Bullough, 1978).

ANA started a certification program for nurse specialists in 1973 to recognize professional achievements and excellence in practice. However, the nurse practitioners needed entry level certification to make them eligible for state certification or licensure, many of the certification examinations have therefore been reoriented to reflect the knowledge base for entry into the specialty.

ANA has long been involved in legislative activities, establishing its first committee for this purpose in 1923. In 1951 a full-time Washington lobbyist was hired. ANA was an early supporter of national health insurance and it has supported a variety of health-related bills since that time. In 1974 it established its own political action committee, the Nurses Coalition for

Action in Politics (N-CAP). In 1984 it supported the Mondale/Ferraro ticket for the Presidency and again in 1992 it took a position in favor of the Democratic ticket, supporting Clinton and Gore because of their stand on health care. The Washington Office publishes a newsletter, *Capital Update,* 24 times a year. *The American Nurse*, the official monthly newsletter of the Association, includes important information about legislation.

Throughout most of its history the individual nurse belonged to three levels: the local, state and national levels of ANA. In 1982 a modified federation structure was adopted, and the individual nurse now belongs to the state association, with the state association belonging to the ANA. Approximately 200,000 registered nurses belong to the ANA, making it the largest nursing organization, although this is only 10% of the nursing work force. The ANA is governed by a house of delegates which meets annually, with a Board of Directors handling business between meetings.

THE NATIONAL LEAGUE FOR NURSING

The National League for Nursing is the oldest existing nursing organization. It was founded in 1893 as the Society of Superintendents of Training Schools for Nurses in United States and Canada, although the Canadian component of the group soon left the Society. Impetus for its establishment came from small group of administrators who met in Chicago at the International Congress of Charities, Correction, and Philanthropy in conjunction with the Worlds Fair. The major focus of the Society was to improve the education of nurses by setting educational standards.

In 1912 the Society changed its name to the National League of Nursing Education. In 1943 the League agreed to admit lay members, and continues to this day to involve dedicated lay persons in its activities. The 1952 amalgamation made it the National League for Nursing, (NLN), which is its current name. This reorganization broadened the functions of the League to include a concern for the quality of nursing care. Originally, this interest was for community health nursing, but recently councils within the league have focused on institutional nursing as well (Bullough, 1991).

The traditional NLN focus on upgrading nursing education is reflected in the organization's current activities including its testing service, consultation services for schools, and the accrediting program for schools of nursing at the master's, baccalaureate, associate, diploma, and practical nursing levels. Four separate councils handle these responsibilities related to nursing education, specifically the Councils of: Baccalaureate and Higher Degree Programs, Associate Degree Programs, Diploma Programs, and Practical Nursing Programs.

In addition to these councils, which represent specific levels of nursing education, there are seven other councils which are focused on other interests: Community Health Services, Nurse Executives, Nursing Informatics, Nursing Centers, Nursing Practice, the Society for Research in Nursing Education, and the Constituent Leagues which brings together 48 local NLN membership groups (Kelly, 1991).

The most important accomplishment of the League in recent years does not, however, center on education. Rather, the league has looked to the importance of nurses in improving nursing care in the community. In 1992 the NLN achieved deemed status for its Community Health Accreditation program (CHAP). This means that home health agencies which are accredited by CHAP will be considered to have met the Government's requirements for participation in Medicare, and will be eligible for reimbursements for services they give clients. Home health care agencies that apply for CHAP accreditation will have to show that they meet minimum standards for quality care. The home health aides they employ will have to demonstrate they meet minimum training requirements, and that they adhere to reasonable standards of patient safety and patients rights. This recognition for nursing as the authority on what constitutes satisfactory nursing care may not sound like a breakthrough, but it is. In the past, the standards used by Medicare were established by other professions or the health care industry (Davis 1992; Fagin, 1992).

AMERICAN ORGANIZATION OF NURSE EXECUTIVES

When ANA took on its collective bargaining functions, the National Labor Relations Act ruled that nurse administrators could not belong to the organization because they would then be sitting on both sides of the bargaining table. The American Hospital Association welcomed the nurse administrators as members, but many still wanted a separate nursing organization, so the American Organization of Nurse Executives was established. Today it serves as the national voice for nurse administrators.

AMERICAN ACADEMY OF NURSING

The American Academy of Nursing was established by ANA in 1973 to provide recognition of professional achievement and excellence. The Academy is made up of nearly 1,000 members, chosen for their professional achievements. It meets annually to discuss nursing issues and to work on studies, reports, and position papers related to major issues.

AMERICAN ASSOCIATION OF COLLEGES OF NURSING

The American Association of Colleges of Nursing (AACN) was established in 1969 as the Conference of Deans of College and University Schools of Nursing. This group was made up of a group of members of the Council of Baccalaureate and Higher Degree Programs of the NLN, who felt that a separate organization was needed to speak for collegiate nursing education particularly in Congress and in federal agencies. The name of the group was changed in 1973 to the American Association of Colleges of Nursing. With the exception of accreditation, which remains an NLN responsibility, many of the functions of the group overlap with those of the NLN Council of Baccalaureate and Higher Degrees.

Throughout the 1970s and 1980s a joint project of the AACN, the ANA Council of Nurse Researchers, and the NLN was to seek the establishment of the National Center for Nursing Research within the National Institutes of Health. This goal was finally accomplished in 1985, and the center has greatly increased the visibility of nursing research and enhanced the funding for nursing studies. Having the Center within its boundaries has also probably helped NIH to broaden its horizons to include a broader range of concerns and more research about women.

THE NATIONAL FEDERATION
OF LICENSED PRACTICAL NURSES

The National Federation of Licensed Practical Nurses (NFLNP) was formed in 1949. It admits only licensed practical nurses (LPNs), licensed vocational nurses (the title used in Texas and California) and student practical nurses. Its goal is to promote better patient care and to speak in behalf of the LPNs. It maintains a Washington office to lobby for LPN issues and cooperates with both ANA and NLN on matters of mutual concern (McGuane & Bullough, 1992).

THE NATIONAL ASSOCIATION FOR PRACTICAL NURSE
EDUCATION AND SERVICE

The National Association for Practical Nurse Education and Service was established in 1944 by a group of nurse educators. The group's first name was the Association of Practical Nurse Schools, and the current title was adopted in 1959. Its focus is on practical nurse education and standards. The group works closely with the Council of Practical Nurse Education of the NLN, and the accreditation function is now handled by the NLN.

THE NATIONAL STUDENT NURSES' ASSOCIATION

The National Student Nurses' Association was established in 1953. Students from any state approved program for registered nurses are eligible for membership. The NSNA speaks to issues in nursing education, health and community affairs, publishes a magazine, *Imprint,* and through its foundation provides scholarships. The state and national meetings are well attended, and the discussions are lively (Nayer, 1987).

COUNCIL OF BLACK NURSES

Organized in the 1970s, the Council of Black Nurses brings Black nurses together for mutual support and political activities. Council members say that ANA has kept its nondiscriminatory pledge made when it took over the functions of the NACGN. However, they still feel the need for a smaller organization made up of people who are concerned with the issue.

REGIONAL ORGANIZATIONS

Five regional organizations focus on nursing education and research and practice. The Western Council on Higher Education in Nursing is the oldest, having been established in the 1960s and reorganized in 1986 as the Western Institute of Nursing (WIN). The Southern Council on Collegiate Education for Nursing (SCCEN) grew out of a Kellogg grant which supported curriculum planning and educational innovation. The Midwest Alliance in Nursing (MAIN) established in 1979 includes sections for nursing service administrators and nursing educators. It has also received Kellogg funding. MAIN served as an organizing body to establish the American Association for the History of Nursing in 1982, although these historians, who are drawn from around the country, are no longer affiliated with MAIN today. The most recently established regional groups are the New England Organization for Nursing (NEON), formed in 1983, and the Mid Atlantic Regional Nursing Association (MARNA). Both of these entities try to bring educators and nursing service administrators together through continuing education and research reports.

NATIONAL ALLIANCE OF NURSE PRACTITIONERS

The National Alliance of Nurse Practitioners was established in 1986, a year after the various groups were brought together by ANA. Its purpose is to promote better health care by supporting nurse practitioners. It includes 12 member organizations. Members must be national in scope or a state group that includes at least 500 members. The Alliance represents 30,000 nurse practitioners, although there is probably some overlap with other organizations. Its actual function is also communication, since, like the NFSNO, decisions on issues are made only with a consensus. However a new ad hoc group, the National Nurse Practitioner Coalition, supported by the Alliance does lobbying in Washington.

SUMMARY AND CONCLUSIONS

Efforts made by nursing leaders in 1952 to amalgamate and limit the number of nursing organizations did not succeed in the long run. Probably the occupation is too large and too diverse for such a limitation, and the variety of organizations that has grown up serves a narrower range of functions. However, it is still possible to see the importance of the two large multipurpose groups. ANA has been instrumental in helping many of the smaller groups get started, and it brought both the specialty organizations and the nurse practitioners together to help them form coalitions. ANA also certifies most of the nurse specialists. NLN for its part has continued to serve the profession by setting educational standards, and more recently in achieving deemed status for its home health accrediting body (CHAP). It seems clear that both large and small organizations are needed. They serve different but important functions for nurses.

TOPICS FOR DISCUSSION

1. Are there too many national nursing organizations? Should nurses try to merge organizations to cut down the number?
2. What makes an organization politically powerful?
3. What type of organization is best for stimulating discussion of clinical problems?
4. Why is the establishment of deemed status for the home health accreditation body of the National League for Nursing an important accomplishment?
5. How can the number of members in the nursing organizations be increased?

REFERENCES

Bullough, B. (1980). *The law and the expanding nursing role.* New York: Appleton-Century-Crofts.

Bullough, V. L., & Bullough, B. (1978). *The care of the sick: The emergence of modern nursing*. New York: Prodist.

Davis, C. K. (1992). Deemed Status for CHAP. *Nursing and Health Care, 13*, 294–295.

Fagin, C. M. (1992). CHAP: America's most achievable health care reform. *Nursing and Health Care, 13*, 283.

Kelly, L. Y. (1991). *Dimensions of professional nursing* (6th ed), New York: Pergamon Press.

McGuane, E. A., & Bullough, B. (1992). Practical nursing: A proud history: A promising future. *The Journal of Practical Nursing, 42*, 13–17.

Nayer, D. (1987). NSNA: How it grew. *Imprint, 34*, 80–86.

3

Nursing Laws and Regulations as They Reflect Societal Issues

Milene A. Megel

Laws are written when sections of the public believe an issue is so important and the perceived need so great that only by legislative directive can the issue be properly addressed. One issue that has forced such legislation has been the protection of the public safety, health, and welfare. Well-known legislative mandates to address this perceived need of the public have been the Social Security Act, National Labor Relations Act, Medicare and Medicaid Act, and the Practice Acts for health professions. All were statutes mandated for the "good" of the people.

This chapter will discuss the impact of three major areas of concern regarding public safety, health, and welfare that have influenced the public's perceived needs regarding nursing and which have demanded the development of statutory legislation, i.e., licensure and testing; an adequate supply of nurses; and quality assurance.

LICENSURE AND TESTING

Nursing has evolved from isolated acts of assisting individuals to a recognized and respected profession that is built upon a sound educational base and which has a defined scope of practice, professional standards, and a code of ethics. Historically, the establishment of nursing as a profession was slow and frustrating because it was tied to the struggle for women's independence and rights. Florence Nightingale is responsible for establishing nursing as one of the first career choices for women. Before Miss Nightingale's time, there was no such thing as professional nursing. By the time of her death in 1910, nursing was a profession that offered women opportunities that were formerly unthinkable.

Nurse Practice Acts

It was not until the early 1900s that the importance of nursing to the public resulted in the passage of laws that attempted to describe what nursing was and who could do it. The first Nurse Practice Acts were developed by North Carolina, New Jersey, New York, and Virginia in 1903 (Roberts, 1954). Over the next 20 years, the states drafted permissive nursing licensure legislation. Permissive licensure regulates only the use of the title and not the nursing actions. Thus, the nurse could not use the title registered professional nurse (RN) unless duly licensed, but could perform many or all of the same nursing actions so long as the nurse did not call himself or herself an RN. New York was the first state to write a mandatory nurse licensing law in 1938, but it did not go into effect until 1947 (Lesnick & Anderson, 1955). By 1953, 15 states had mandatory licensing legislation, and many had certain statutory exceptions. The legislation for Nurse Practice Act amendments to make licensure mandatory was basically the result of actions and lobbying by the American Nurses Associations of each state. Table 3.1 identifies the dates of enactment of licensure laws by each state (American Nurses Association, 1940, personal communications with boards of nursing staff members of Virgin Islands, W. Garfield; Wyoming, T. Nisbet; Texas, M. Majek; & Kansas, J. Pucci; June 1992).

Enactment of the licensure laws included regulations for licensure by examination. Individual state boards developed questions and administered and graded the written and practical examinations of candidates. The state boards expressed early concerns about the use of such nonstandardized tests. Studies and board experiences indicated that the practical examinations lacked validity. The state-prepared essay examinations were time-consuming to develop and score and were also of questionable validity in licensure decisions.

State Board Test Pool Examinations

A report by the subcommittee on Tests of the National League for Nursing Education Committee on State Board Problems, read at the League's 1939 convention, proposed the pooling of test items by states and the development of an objective machine-scorable test. The first State Board Test Pool Examination (SBTPE) for RNs was officially released in January 1944 and consisted of 13 tests in the areas of anatomy and physiology; chemistry; communicable disease nursing; obstetric nursing; pharmacology; psychiatric nursing; social foundation; and surgical nursing (National League for Nursing, 1985). Twenty-two states and the District of Columbia used all or parts of the examination in 1944, and by 1950 all

TABLE 3.1 Dates State Licensure Laws Were Enacted

1903	1904	1905
03/03—NC	03/25—MD	02/27—IN
04/01—NJ		03/03—CA
04/27—NY		04/12—CO
05/14—VA		07/01—CT
1907	**1908**	**1909**
02/09—DC	01/08—MN	02/18—WY
02/19—WV	03/11—DE	03/02—OK
03/12—IA		03/03—WA
08/22—GA		03/10—NH
05/02—IL		03/24—NB
		03/28—TX
		05/01—PA
		05/05—MO
		06/01—MI
1910	**1911**	**1912**
02/23—SC	01/28—VT	05/12—RI
04/29—MA	03/09—ID	07/12—LA
	03/15—OR	
	04/05—TN	
	06/17—WI	
1913	**1914**	**1915**
02/12—KS	03/01—MS	03/09—ND
03/03—MT	03/13—KY	03/18—ME
03/05—AR		05/03—OH
06/07—FL		08/06—AL
1917	**1921**	**1923**
01/24—SD	06/10—AZ	02/13—NM
04/03—HI		03/20—NV
07/17—UT		
1930	**1941**	**1952**
05/15—PR	03/27—AK	08/08—VI

states used the SBTPE for licensing purposes. Table 3.2 identifies the year each state began to use the SBTPE, dates of withdrawal, and return (National League for Nursing, 1972).

Hawaii and Alaska began to use the SBTPE in 1946 and 1953, respectively, followed by Guam in 1960 and the Virgin Islands in 1963. Seven Canadian provinces administered the SBTPE until 1971: Alberta—1953; British Columbia—1949; Manitoba—1955; Newfoundland—1961; Nova Scotia—1955; Prince Edward Island—1956; Quebec—1959; and Saskatchewan—1956 (National League for Nursing, 1985).

The development of the SBTPE soon demonstrated that a clearinghouse was needed by state boards to obtain the information needed to produce

TABLE 3.2 Enrollment Dates of States Using the SBTPE

1944—AL, CT, DC, FL, GA, LO, MA, MI, MS, NE, NJ, NM, NY, NC, ND, OR, SD, TN, VT, VA, WA, WI, WY

1945—KS, MD, MO
   Withdrew: FL, MA, NY, NC, VA

1946—AZ, AR, CA, IA, ME, MN, OH, PA, SC, UT
   Withdrew: WA, WY

1947—DE, IN, NH, RI
   Rejoined: NC, WA, WY

1948—CO
   Rejoined: VA

1949—ID, IL, KY, MS, NV, OK, TX

1950—WV
   Rejoined: FL, MA, NY

test items. A Bureau of State Boards of Nursing began to operate out of American Nurses Association headquarters. Over the next 30 years discussion regarding a potential conflict of interest developed between the Bureau (later the Council) of State Boards and the professional Association. On June 5, 1978, the American Nurses Association Council of State Boards of Nursing voted to withdraw and form the National Council of State Boards of Nursing, Inc. (National Council of State Boards of Nursing, 1990).

National Council Licensure Examination

The National Council of State Boards of Nursing, Inc. (NCSBN) is a group composed of members and executive secretaries/directors of boards of nursing of the United States and territories. The first National Council Licensure Examination NCLEX was given to nurse candidates in 1982. It continued to be a paper and pencil examination until in 1990, the NCSBN Delegate Assembly in Chicago, Illinois, voted to develop a Computerized Adaptive Test (CAT) for licensure to be implemented in 1994. The move to computer testing required statutory and regulatory changes by states to remove language that addressed "paper and pencil examinations" and that required applicants to take the same test on the same test dates. The CAT examination will be tailored to assess the applicant's competence by having the computer select the difficulty of a successive item based-upon the response of the candidate to the previous test item. A three-year implementation schedule was projected to allow states the time to make the necessary statutory changes.

AN ADEQUATE SUPPLY OF NURSES

The demand for nurses has always outdistanced the supply. The need for nurses grew as medicine became more sophisticated, technology advanced, new surgical techniques were developed, and diagnostic tests increased in complexity. Every war demanded qualified nurses to provide the needed care. At the end of every war nurses have been released from duty and returned to civilian nursing practice, but there were never "enough" nurses.

The first national health survey was conducted by the U.S. Public Health Service in 1935 and 1936. For the first time a nationwide picture of the country's health was available. Presidential commissions began to study the delivery of health care and to predict the number of professionals needed in order to provide the level of health care demanded by the public. The President's Commission to Study the Health Needs of the Nation, appointed by President Truman, published five volumes in 1952 (Jensen, 1959). The reports indicated that the nation needed more nurses to meet the demand for nursing services. Federal legislation providing grant monies for applicants to nursing schools was passed, which encouraged student enrollment. Government support for nurses and nursing programs expanded through 1960 and 1970 and then maintained a consistent level of support.

Foreign Recruitment

Early licensure statutes had strict regulations regarding the age of nurse candidates and citizenship requirements. As the demand for nurses grew, the prerequisite requirements diminished. In 1952, at least 23 states reported a citizenship or declaration of intent requirement, and 16 required a minimum age of 21 (American Nurses Association, 1952). By 1962, no state required a minimum age of 21 (American Nurses Association, 1962). Presently, only one State, Kansas, has a citizenship requirement (National Council of State Boards of Nursing, 1990). The increased demand for nurses caused employers to look for other avenues to fill their needs, and an interest in recruiting foreign nurses developed. In the late 1960s, the federal government enacted the Immigration and Naturalization Service Regulations, these allowed foreign nurses to enter the U.S. on H-1 visas to work in states that issued temporary permits, pending taking and passing the examination for licensure. Health care institutions began to recruit nurses from foreign countries to fill vacancies. Initially, recruitment efforts were directed to English-speaking countries, Canada and the Philippines, but gradually extended to countries where English was not the primary language. Between 1969 and 1977, approximately 75,000 foreign nurses entered the USA to seek employment as RNs.

The failure rate on the licensure examination for foreign-educated nurses was four times that of U.S.-educated nurses. In 1975, the Department of Health, Education and Welfare (DHEW) estimated that almost 50% of the nurses educated in other countries never succeeded in becoming licensed in the U.S. In June 1965, DHEW convened a conference of nursing organizations and governmental agencies to discuss the problems experienced by foreign-educated nurses in meeting U.S. legal, educational and examination requirements. At the conclusion of the conference, there was a consensus of opinion that a central agency should be established for all matters relating to immigration of foreign nurses and that a pre-immigration/prelicensing examination be developed (Division of Nursing, 1975).

Commission on Graduates of Foreign Nursing Schools

The American Nurses' Association and the National League of Nursing sponsored the formation of the Commission on Graduates of Foreign Nursing Schools (CGFNS) and supplied money to establish the commission, which was incorporated as an autonomous, nonprofit organization in Pennsylvania in 1977.

Immediately, DHEW awarded a contract to CGFNS to carry out an "Investigation into the Readiness of Graduates of Foreign Nursing Schools to Meet Licensure Requirements in the USA" (Herwitz, 1979). An examination was developed to test nursing theory and practice in the fields of medical, surgical, obstetric, pediatric, and psychiatric nursing, and was first administered on October 4, 1978. The examination also tested English language comprehension, vocabulary, and sentence structure. At the completion of the study, recommendations included:

foreign nurse graduates must achieve a passing grade on the CGFNS examination in order to qualify for a Labor Certificate and an Occupational Preference Visa;
state boards of nursing should require the CGFNS as a prerequisite to taking the SBTPE in any state; and
the Joint Commission on Accreditation of Hospitals should require accredited hospitals to accept for employment only foreign nurse graduates who have passed the CGFNS/SBTPE examinations.

In August 1979, the Immigration and Naturalization Service proposed federal regulations requiring nonimmigrant professional nurses to pass the CGFNS examination in order to qualify for the H-1 Visa (Federal Register, 1979). Since 1980, an Occupational Preference Visa has been granted only to CGFNS certificate holders or nurses holding a full and unrestricted license in their state of employment. The 1989 Immigration Nursing Relief Act continued the requirement, but placed stipulations on the employers of nurses on temporary occupational visas and changed the visa designation from H-1 to H-1a. The Department of Labor issues work permits to foreign educated nurses who hold CGFNS certificates (Immigration Nursing Relief Act, 1989).

In 1977, Wyoming became the first state to require the CGFNS certificate. Within ten years, 40 states, Washington, D.C., Guam, and the Virgin Islands had similar statutes. Ohio legislation passed in 1991. In a move designed to increase access to nursing, in 1990 New York legislatively removed the CGFNS requirement for admission to the licensing examination, but maintained the requirement for issuance of a limited permit. Presently, 12 states that do not require the CGFNS certificate as a prerequisite to take the NCLEX: Alaska, Arkansas, California, Colorado, Florida, Georgia, Maryland, Michigan, Minnesota, Nebraska, New York and South Carolina (Commission on Graduates of Foreign Nursing Schools Survey, 1987–1990).

Despite the perpetual belief held by the public that there was a shortage of nurses, there was no systematic collection of data regarding the number and characteristics of the nurse population until *Facts About Nursing* began to be published by the American Nurses Association in 1935. The data were supplied by nursing groups and boards of nursing. Its major flaw regarding the number of nurses licensed in each state was (and continues to be) that one nurse can be counted many times. A nurse is not limited to holding only one license in one state, as is true in the case of a driver's license, so holding licensure in multiple states allows for multiple counting of one nurse.

The NCSBN announced in November 1991 that the Organization was the recipient of a grant from the Robert Wood Johnson Foundation to study the feasibility of establishing a National Nurse Information System (NIS). An 11-month feasibility study was designed to evaluate approaches to resolving several issues that affect on the establishment and maintenance of an NIS.

One aspect of the study was to evaluate the ability to compile an unduplicated list of RNs licensed to practice in one or more states. The development of a computer-based, national NIS composed of unduplicated master lists of individuals licensed as RNs and/or licensed practical nurses (LPNs) would provide a means for obtaining a count of and the geographic distribution of individuals holding an active license to practice nursing in the U.S. In addition to the Robert Wood Johnson Foundation grant, the NIS project was funded by the Division of Nursing and the American Nurses Association (National Council awarded grant, 1991).

Advanced Practitioners

As the demand for health care has increased, so too has the need for highly educated health care providers. Longer life expectancy has resulted in an aging population who have multiple chronic illnesses and diseases that require more surgical interventions and complex care. The need for more complex care has increasingly been met by nurses who have advanced their education by becoming nurse practitioners, clinical specialists, and nurse anesthetists. Nurse midwives are increasing in numbers to meet the needs of women who desire an alternative to the medical management of childbirth. States are now attempting to regulate the practice of advanced practitioners. The NCSBN suggests that states consider some of the following criteria when selecting an appropriate level of regulation for professional practice:

the risk of harm to the consumer;
the specialized education skills and abilities required for the professional
    practice;
level of autonomy;
scope of practice;
economic impact;
alternatives to regulation; and
a determination of the least restrictive regulation consistent with public
    safety (National Council of State Boards of Nursing, 1992).

There are four levels of regulation used by the different states: credential recognition, registry placement, certification, and licensure. The NCSBN (1986) originally published a position paper that encouraged states to certify advanced practice through national association certification examinations, similar to the method used by the medical profession. Only six years later, a draft paper prepared for the 1992 Delegate Assembly proposed that advanced practice be regulated through licensure (National Council of State Boards of Nursing, 1992). The paper was approved by the 1993 Delegate Assembly despite strong oppoisition from the American Nurses' Association and other advanced practice nursing groups.

QUALITY ASSURANCE

The recipient of health care services has historically trusted health care providers to be current and up-to-date on health care knowledge and practices. In the 1960s, a consumer movement came into prominence, and considerable emphasis was placed on the responsibility of health professionals to provide appropriate care to the citizenry, particularly minority members and the poor. Health professionals were expected to act in the public good. Consumer groups began to review health care outcomes and to demand accountability. The identification of deficiencies in the health care delivery system initiated the development of plans for improvement.

Continuing Education

The 1970s pushed the consumer movement into an era of accountability and sparked an interest in the competency of health professionals. Professional associations began to stress voluntary continuing education for members and to establish recordkeeping mechanisms that allowed members to keep track of the continuing education units that they earned.

The next step was mandatory continuing education. The nursing associations responsible for certification of advanced practice were the first to require continuing education for recertification as a continuing competency mechanism. The first states to legislate mandatory continuing education for RNs were California, Kansas, and Minnesota in 1978 (American Nurses' Association, 1982–1983). In the next 10 years, 20 states passed legislation that required varying amounts of continuing education in order to be reregistered or relicensed. Then the legislation appeared to lose the early momentum; states found the requirement to be costly to implement. Despite the cost and lack of validity studies to determine the impact of such legislation, the public continued to view it in a positive light. By 1990, four more states had enacted legislation for continuing competency mechanisms in statute and pending implementation dates of 1992 for Delaware and Texas; and 1994 for Louisiana and Ohio (Wise, 1992).

Peer Assistance Programs

Substance abuse, which began as a symbol of rebellion for the youth of the 1960s, had become a growing concern among professionals in the 1990s. The extent of substance abuse by health professionals is unknown, but the proportion of professional discipline cases involving substance abuse has been increasing. Support programs have been developed by state governments and state professional associations; however, little data has been published regarding the numbers of professionals entering and leaving the programs, or the rate of recidivism.

Most states provide some services to impaired nurses, ranging from referrals to appropriate agencies (42 states), education (46), intervention (21), and re-entry monitoring (19) to a hotline (11), but only 13 states have enacted diversion legislation (American Nurses Association, 1991). A

Professional Assistance Program, such as that passed by the New York legislature in 1988, provides the impaired professional with immunity from disciplinary action if there was no evidence of patient harm and the professional voluntarily entered a treatment program. Application to the program required temporary surrender of the license and a consent to appropriate monitoring while in the program. By 1992, nurses made up the majority of professional participants in the New York program, but the number was small compared to the total number of licensees in the State (State Education Department, 1990–1991). The New York legislature has considered eliminating the mandatory surrender as a means to encourage increased participation of licensed professionals in the program.

FUTURE ISSUES FOR LEGISLATION AFFECTING NURSES

The public will continue to be concerned over its health, safety and welfare; however, the emphasis will vary between costs, services and providers. Clients will be more educated and aware of their needs through modern communication channels and will continue to demand "quality" in the health care delivery system and an adequate number of caregivers. This heightened interest in health care delivery will be the force behind a "cookbook" managed care approach to health care. Successful, documented, and proven health care will be expected by every health care recipient and at a reasonable expenditure of time, money, and medical resources. Standards of care and standards of practice will be redefined to form a common basis for deciding which health care providers and health care plans are cost-effective and successful. State legislation will be needed to alter professional practice acts to reflect these changes.

States will need to determine how advanced practitioners will be recognized. In a survey of NCSBN member boards in November 1991, 13 states licensed one or more categories of advanced practitioners (nurse anesthetists, nurse midwives, nurse practitioners, and clinical nurse specialists), 22 states certified one or more categories, and 19 states used other methods of recognition (V. Sheets, personal communication, June 14, 1992). The interstate mobility of advanced practitioners will be potentially threatened if there is no agreement between states on the process of credentialing advanced practitioners. This will be a major issue for states in the next five years.

There will be increased interest in holding down health care costs by delegating more duties to the next lower level of health personnel and by expanding the existing roles of professionals. Surveys of boards of nursing have indicated that in the last few years, 25 states have proposed legislation that allows nurses to delegate additional tasks that previously were considered professional nursing to LPNs, and 26 have proposed legislation to expand the role of the RN (Practice Committee Report, 1991). The expansion of the professional roles and the authorized downward delegation of nursing acts to other licensed professionals provides the public with additional safeguards. If care is delivered by a professional, states have rules defining unprofessional conduct and a disciplinary process dedicated to the investigation and prosecution of negligent or incompetent health care providers. This process provides the public with a means of obtaining "justice" for professional wrongdoing. Unlicensed personnel do not have a comparable disciplinary process, and cases of negligent care by unlicensed personnel must be litigated on an individual basis by the State Attorney General.

The increased use of unlicensed personnel may eventually stimulate the public's interest in government regulation of the actions of such personnel in the health field. Present-day assistive health care personnel have the potential to become the licensed or certified health care providers of the future. After all, nursing evolved in a not too dissimilar manner.

States face many legislative challenges in the ensuing years regarding the health care delivery system. Consumer demands will control the direction of legislative initiatives. The public health, safety, and welfare will always be a driving force.

TOPICS FOR DISCUSSION

1. Discuss whether or not you think nurses who practice advanced nursing should be required to have a second license?
2. Which of the four categories of advanced nursing (nurse anesthetists, nurse practitioner, nurse midwife and clinical nurse specialist) should have plenary authority to prescribe?
3. Should practical nursing programs be extended in length and include more knowledge and skills to create a more "advanced" licensed practical nurse?
4. Do you think continuing education for nurses should be mandatory?
5. Are there any nursing tasks that you think could be taught to unlicensed individuals that are not now taught to unlicensed individuals? Discuss your rationale for your decisions.
6. Should nurses not educated in the United States be required to speak and understand English as a prerequisite to U.S. licensure?

REFERENCES

American Nurses Association. (1940). *A digest of nurse practice acts and board rules*. New York: Author.

American Nurses Association. (1952). *Facts about nursing*. Kansas City, MO: Author.

American Nurses Association. (1962). *Facts about nursing*. Kansas City, MO: Author.

American Nurses Association. (1982–1983).*Facts about nursing*. Kansas City, MO: Author.

American Nurses Association. (1991). *Addictions and psychological dysfunctions in nursing: The profession's response to the problem*. Kansas City, MO: Author.

Commission on Graduates of Foreign Nursing Schools. (1990). *Board of nursing survey on state regulations regarding foreign educated nurses*. Philadelphia, PA: Author.

Division of Nursing. Public Hrealth Services, U.S. Department of Health and Human Sciences. (1975). *Conference on immigration of graduates of foreign nursing schools*. Washington, D.C.: U.S. Government Printing Office.

Nonimmigrant alien (H-1) nurses; proposed examination requirement. (1979). *Federal Register, 44*,(169). Washington, DC: U.S. Government Printing Office.

Herwitz, A. (1979). *Investigation into the readiness of graduates of foreign nursing schools to meet licensure requirements in the United States* (DHEW, HRA 231-77-00078). Washington, D.C.: U.S. Government Printing Office.

Immigration Nursing Relief Act of 1989. One hundred first congress 101, 13 U.S.C. (H.R. 1507 & H.R. 2111, serial no. 13) 3259. Washington, DC: U.S. Government Printing Office.

Jensen, D. (1959). *History and trends of professional nursing*. St. Louis: Mosby.

Lesnick, M., & Anderson, B. (1955). *Nursing practice and the law* (2nd ed.). Philadelphia: Lippincott.

National Council Awarded Grant from Robert Wood Johnson Foundation to Study Feasibility of Establishing a National Nurse Information System. (1991). *Issues, 12*, 5.

National Council of State Boards of Nursing. (1986).*Position paper on the licensure of advanced nursing practice*. Chicago: Author.

National Council of State Boards of Nursing. (1990). *Orientation manual*. Profiles of Member Boards. Chicago: Author.

National Council of State Boards of Nursing. (1992).*Position paper on the licensure of advanced nursing practice*. Chicago: Author.

National League for Nursing. (1972). *Chronological list of significant events relating to council activities and the state board test pool*. A National League for nursing document presented to the Council of State Boards of nursing in April. New York: Author. (Unpublished manuscript)

National League for Nursing. (1985). *An historical survey of the test services of the NLN* (Pub. 17-777). New York: Author.

Practice Committee Report. (1991). *Delegate assembly agenda book*. Chicago: National Council State Boards of Nursing, Inc.

Roberts, M. (1954). *American nursing: History and interpretation*. New York: MacMillan.

State Education Department. (1990–91). *Office of the professions: Annual report*. Albany, NY: Author.

Wise, P. (1992). State and association continuing education requirements. *Journal of Continuing Education, 23*, 3–5.

4

Overview of Legal Issues for Nurses

Andrew Feldman and Joy Feldman

The field of nursing has come far during the twentieth century. Today, nursing is indisputably a profession, founded upon an ever-growing body of knowledge with standardized educational credentials, and licensed by state law which sets forth the scope of practice for the profession. As nursing practice evolves to roles of increased independence, individual responsibility and liability also evolve and attach to that independence. The result has been an increase in nurses being individually named as defendants in lawsuits.

The purpose of this chapter is to introduce readers to basic legal issues involved in nursing practice. Understanding one's legal obligations is fundamental to avoiding the pitfalls of malpractice and professional misconduct. The resulting benefit to the patients is as significant as is the avoidance of the trauma of lawsuits for the nurse.

The chapter first sets forth theories under which a nurse may be held liable for malpractice. The categories of nursing errors that most frequently result in malpractice litigation are then explored. Next, the significance of the medical record is discussed; nursing entries into medical records are critical contributions to document the health care rendered. Facts reflected there may either establish a case against or exonerate professionals accused of negligence. Governmental standards and regulations affecting nursing practice are then summarized. Last, specifics on how nurses may avoid malpractice is explored. The most common errors that implicate nurses in lawsuits are discussed.

THEORIES OF LIABILITY

Negligence: The Standard of Care

The term malpractice has dreaded overtones. Nurses and other health care providers should not feel that the term is directed solely toward them. Malpractice, as a rule of law, actually refers to alleged failure on the part of any professional to render services with the degree of care, diligence, and precaution that a member of the same profession under similar circumstances would render to prevent injury to someone else. The "doing" or "failing to do," that which any reasonable and prudent fellow professional would do under the same or similar circumstances, constitutes a cause of action in malpractice, when that results in injury to someone else. Professionals who are subject to malpractice claims include nurses, physicians, architects, engineers, lawyers, and insurance brokers, to name only a few.

The Individual's Duty of Care

A nurse must realize that as a professional she or he has certain legal obligations to the patient. Once a nurse/patient relationship has been established, legal obligations arise for both parties. A nurse-patient relationship, in effect, is a contract for professional services. Additionally, the relationship, itself, creates an obligation for the nurse, called "the duty of care." On the patient's part, entering the relationship conveys consent to be treated by the nurse. The complementarity gives rise to several possible bases of patient claims of malpractice. Although the nurse is practicing nursing, not medicine, nursing practice is included in the realm of "medical malpractice" under the law.

The law relating to a medical malpractice claims against nurses differs little from state to state. For a patient to establish a successful malpractice claim against a nurse, the following prerequisites have to be established:

1. A relationship has to exist between the patient and the nurse;
2. A duty has to be established as a result of that relationship;
3. There has to be a breach of duty owed by the nurse to the patient, i.e., an error or an omission on the part of the nurse; and
4. There has to be an injury to the patient which was proximately related to the error or omission (breach of duty) by the nurse.

The legal standard of care is based on what a reasonable and prudent nurse would have done in similar circumstances. That set of actions is generally determined from the following sources:

1. testimony from an expert nurse or doctor;
2. the policies and procedures of the institution;
3. state and federal regulations that are applicable to the care and treatment rendered;
4. standards of professional associations; and
5. the current professional literature relative to the care and treatment rendered to patients.

The court will generally charge a jury in a malpractice case pending against a nurse with the following law:

> A nurse's responsibility is the same whether or not he or she is paid for their services. By undertaking to perform a medical service, the nurse does not, nor does the law require that the nurse guarantee a good result. The nurse is only liable for negligence.
>
> A nurse cannot be found negligent unless he or she is found to have breached his or her duty to the patient.
>
> "Duty" is any action necessary in or appropriate to one's occupation or position. The nurse's duty is based on standards of care that have been discussed and also as set forth in state and federal statutes, rules and regulations, and court cases.
>
> The law recognizes that there are differences in the abilities of nurses, just as there are in the abilities of people engaged in other activities. To practice his or her profession, a nurse is not required to be possessed of the extraordinary knowledge and ability that belongs to a few individuals of rare endowments. However, the nurse is required to keep abreast of the times and to practice in accordance with the approved methods and means of treatment in general use. The standard to which the nurse is held is measured by the degree of knowledge and ability of the average nurse in good standing in the community where he or she practices.
>
> In performing a medical service, the nurse is obligated to use his or her best judgment and to use reasonable care in the exercise of that knowledge and ability. The rule requiring the nurse to use his or her best judgment does not make the nurse liable for a mere error in judgment, provided the nurse does what he or she thinks is best after careful examination. The nurse, like any professional, is allowed to make an honest error in judgment. The rule of reasonable care does not require the exercise of the highest degree of care: it requires only that degree of care that a reasonably prudent nurse would exercise under the same circumstances. This rule allows for the fact that medicine is not an exact science, and that latitude should be given to the health care provider to exercise discretion in treatment decisions.
>
> If a patient sustains injury while undergoing medical care and that injury results from a breach of duty by the nurse, whether

that be through lack of knowledge or ability, or from the nurse's failure to exercise reasonable care or to use his or her best judgment, then the nurse is responsible for the injuries that result from the nurse's acts." (Douthwaite, 1987, pp. 340–341)

Vicarious Liability—Respondeat Superior

"The Doctrine of Respondeat Superior" has been asserted by injured parties in an effort to impose liability on hospitals. Respondeat superior means "let the master answer."

In general, this theory allows an injured party to recover from the individual's employer. For example, nurses and other attendants at the hospital who are negligent in performing their duties, or fail to perform their duties, make their employer liable.

Because of the principle of respondeat superior, hospitals, as employers of nurses, are viewed as principal targets for the recovery of damages because of their perceived economic resources. The facilities where the nurses are employed become the target defendants because of this doctrine, and the facilities at which the nurses work have a vested interest in making certain that their personnel are qualified to perform the duties assigned to them.

Informed Consent

A bedrock principle in American law is the right to be free of bodily interference from anther person. This right to "autonomy" is an aspect of liberty, and is guaranteed by the U.S. Constitution through the 14th amendment of the Bill of Rights. Unwanted touching is assault, and the threat of assault is battery. Invasion of one's territory or space without consent is trespass. These violations of one's liberty interests are "torts" for which American law provides remedy through civil court action, and damages in the form of money awards.

Our cultural value on the individual's right to control what happens to his/her own body is constitutionally protected such that unwanted medical care or treatment, regardless of whether it is "well-meant" or "in the best interests" of the patient, is actionable in tort. The facts of an often cited case, and the court's decision, illustrate this principle vividly. Mary Schloendorff was admitted to the hospital in 1908 suffering with a stomach malady. She later testified that the doctor sought and obtained her consent to perform an "ether examination" in order to diagnosis her difficulty, but that she notified her physician that she did not want to undergo an operation. During the ether examination, a tumor was found and removed, according to her testimony, without her consent or knowledge.

Mary Schloendorff developed gangrene of the arm following the procedure, for which some fingers were amputated; she then sued the hospital. The case was litigated up to the highest court of the State of New York.

The final opinion by Chief Judge Benjamin Cardozo of the New York State Court of Appeals, stated: "The wrong complained of is not merely negligence. It is trespass. Every human being of adult years and sound mind has the right to determine what shall be done with his own body; and a surgeon who performs an operation without his patient's consent commits an assault, for which he is liable in damages. This is true except in cases of emergency where the patient is unconscious and where it is necessary to operate before consent can be obtained." *Schloendorff v. New York Hospital* (1914).

The legal system places the burden of giving an Informed Consent upon the physician, and requires the physician to communicate to the patient adequate information so that the patient can knowledgeably decide whether or not to go forward with a proposed diagnostic or operative procedure. The need for a patient's consent is based upon the fundamental, legal, medical, and moral principle that a medical procedure should not be performed without a patient's consent. That consent must be based upon the patient being fully informed.

Although the law in each state regarding Informed Consent may vary slightly, generally, a physician performing an operation or diagnostic procedure, is under a duty to explain, in terms understandable to the patient, the following:

1. What he/she proposes to do;
2. The reason for the operation or procedure; and
3. What the risks and benefits will be; what the alternatives are; and what to expect if the procedure or alternatives are not done.

The doctor is under a duty to explain all the facts so that the patient may give his or her consent based on awareness of:

1. His or her existing physical condition;
2. The purpose of, and the advantage of submitting to the operation or procedure;
3. The risk to his or her health or life which the operation or procedure may impose;
4. The risks involved if no operation or procedure is performed; and
5. The available alternative operations or procedures, and the risks and disadvantages involved in them.

An adult patient who is conscious and competent has the right to refuse to permit any medical or surgical procedure, and a competent patient's refusal must be honored. This is true whether the refusal is grounded upon a doubt that the contemplated procedure will be successful, upon a concern about the probable or possible results of the procedure, upon a lack of confidence in the surgeon who recommends it, or upon religious belief. Furthermore, situations can arise before treatment has actually begun in which the patient specifically prohibits a procedure or technique that might be necessary during treatment. In the event of such a refusal, the health care provider has an obligation to treat the patient and provide only such services or procedures that are within the limits stated by the patient. It must be emphasized that a patient has the right to control his or her own medical destiny, even though the medical treatment may be considered necessary.

An incompetent patient, or minor, may have a designated legal representative, or parent, give a substituted consent. When there is no designated representative, a petition can be made by the court to obtain an Order for an appropriate representative to authorize the procedure.

The nurse's role with regard to obtaining the consent is generally ministerial, wherein the nurse may take the form to the patient for signature, and may witness the signing of consent. The actual responsibility for obtaining consent is the legal obligation of the physician performing the procedure or treatment. A physician meets his or her legal obligation by disclosing the necessary information to the patient. Although it is not necessary that the physician obtain a written consent from the patient, it is advisable that the patient's consent be in fact documented. In the absence of a written and signed consent, a physician could not later prove that (s)he obtained the patient's Informed Consent.

The nurse has no legal duty or authority to inform patients, or to assess their level of understanding regarding risks, benefits, and alternatives. Generally, it is the practice in many hospitals for the nurses to obtain the patient's signature acknowledging that the patient is going to be undergoing a specific surgical procedure or invasive procedure. That is not to be confused with the physician's obligation to obtain the patient's Informed Consent.

It is not the duty of the nurse to insure that the Informed Consent process has taken place. However, the nurse should be aware of the fact that the Joint Commission on Accreditation of Hospitals (JCAH) requires the hospital to establish a protocol that clearly specifies responsibilities for completing the Informed Consent process. It also requires that:

1. Evidence of the patient's Informed Consent be documented in the medical record; and
2. Nursing staff members alert the hospital to any indication of a patient's confusion or lack of awareness regarding treatment about to be given to him or her.

If the nurse determines that the physician has not discussed the surgery with the patient, then the nurse should notify the appropriate personnel in the hospital, as well as the physician, so that there is no question that the patient understands the nature of the procedure, the surgical risks, benefits, and alternatives. The nurse witnessing the patient's signature on the consent agreement does not attest to the fact that an Informed Consent was in fact given by the patient, or the patient's level of understanding. Rather, the act of witnessing attests to the fact that the signature of the person consenting is authentically that of the patient. That is important, because only the patient him- or herself may consent to or refuse his or her own treatment. Only in special circumstances may someone other than the patient have legal authority to consent or refuse on behalf of the patient.

Invasion of Privacy

The Right to Refuse Treatment

The trespass found in the case of Mary Schloendorff underscores the role of privacy in relation to a person and his/her right to accept or refuse even "needed" medical care. The fundamental right to privacy and autonomy protected by Informed Consent has taken on increasing importance in recent times. The same privacy right that underlies the Informed Consent requirement also gives foundation to the individual's absolute right to refuse medical care, even if that refusal will result in the illness, demise, or death of the person refusing.

Advances in medical technology have resulted in increasing ambiguity between life and death. Knowing when to withdraw life-sustaining treatment, or when to withhold invasive procedures or life support, rests on recognizing when intervention holds hope for restoring life, and when, in fact, death is inevitable or indeed, already happening. Further, what constitutes "life" worthy of sustaining varies with values and morals unique to each person. These individual differences of profound importance do not lend themselves easily to settling with a rule of law.

The societal value placed on life and its preservation has long supported unquestioned reliance on medical interventions that restore function or at least postpone death for a while. As medical care and technology have become increasingly capable of forestalling death and preserving some measure of life functions, our society has created ethical, moral, economic, and legal dilemmas.

Despite the extensive tradition and legal protection of the right to privacy, autonomy, and freedom from unwanted interference, those personal rights have historically not received protection for the patient who becomes unable to consider the options and communicate refusal of treatment. In clinical care settings, decision making has traditionally been the province of the physician, with more or less consultation with the patient and/or family members. Particularly in circumstances where the patient's ability to make decisions has been limited, for whatever reason, decisions have been made in his stead by the one(s) in control nearby.

The right to refuse medical care is not new in American law. What is new is the protection of this right past the loss of decision making capacity, through state statutes that began to emerge during the 1980s. High profile court cases dealing with patient's rights to forgo life-sustaining measures both highlighted and publicized the tension between competing values and ethics. State legislatures began to create guidelines for the increasingly vexing problems of when, how much, and who shall decide about treatment measures.

Competency vs. Capability

The right of a person to control his own body is a fundamental societal concept, protected in the common law throughout our nation's history. It is also fundamental that a person does not lose his/her civil rights unless (s)he has been adjudicated "incompetent" by a court, in which case the court then appoints a Guardian over the "incompetent" in order to protect the person's (civil) rights. Accordingly, a person whose clinical condition impairs his/her thought processes or level of consciousness, nonetheless retains legal competence and the corollary constitutional right to make decisions concerning his/her own body. For example, a diagnosed psychotic still has the right to refuse treatment (qualified only by whether (s)he is a danger to self or others); a disoriented person with Alzheimer's still has the right to refuse treatment; even well-meaning others do not have the legal right to substitute as decision makers unless they do so pursuant to state law that authorizes the substitution.

This is a critical concept for nurses and other health care workers to grasp. The right to consent to treatment and the right to refuse treatment belongs to the patient. This is not a change in the law, but a departure from traditional medical practice that was not supported by law. Regardless of others' perceptions of whether the patient is "competent" to make health care decisions, it is the patient's exclusive right to exercise, unless the patient has been adjudged incompetent by a court, or unless a state law authorizes a substitute decision maker to be appointed. A few states have begun to enact legislation to allow substitute decisionmaking for patients in circumstances such as persistent vegetative state and advanced terminal illness.

Advance Medical Directives

So important is the protection of the right to consent to or refuse treatment that legal measures have emerged by which these rights can be protected, should the capacity to exercise them be lost as a person's clinical condition declines in the future. Many states have "Living Will" statutes wherein a person can direct what (s)he would want done under various circumstances if (s)he became unable to make or communicate decisions about treatment. Some states have enacted Health Care Proxy laws, wherein a person can designate another to act as an agent on his/her behalf. A person thereby empowers their agent to make any decision for them that they would make themselves if they had the capacity.

Enactment of the federal amendment to OBRA (the Omnibus Budget Reconciliation Act), known as "The Patient Self-Determination Act," effective December 1, 1991, highlighted the importance of this emergent protection. The Act is limited to health care providers who participate in Medicare and Medicaid, only because the principal of federalism preserves to the states and the people powers not granted to the federal government under the Constitution. Clearly, the Patient Self-Determination Act was meant by Congress to reach and affect health care delivery to the limits of federal authority.

The Patient Self-Determination Act requires health care providers to:

1. Inform every adult, both orally and in writing, of their right under state law to make decisions concerning medical care, including their right to refuse medical or surgical treatment, and their right to make advance medical directives;
2. Have and provide written statements of policies of the health care provider concerning the implementation of the patient's rights in the health care decision making process;
3. Have a written statement affirming that the facility will not condition provision of care or discriminate in any way based on whether or not the patient has executed an advance directive;
4. Document the patient's medical record, whether or not (s)he has made an advance directive;
5. Have a written statement insuring compliance by the facility with the requirements of the state law respecting advance directives; and
6. Conduct programs of education for the facility staff and the community on medical and legal issues concerning advance directives.

It is noteworthy that the 1990s ushered in such a sweeping federal measure to ensure protection of patient's rights. By placing the onus on health care providers to educate not only their patients but also the community about their rights to their own health care decision making, Congress made clear its intent: no longer does the health care provider (store owner) decide what the patient (the customer) needs and will get. Mandated through OBRA, health care providers' compliance will be monitored through state health department surveys that allow continuing licensure.

These measures satisfy in part the need for clarification over who owns responsibility for making decisions that

1. impact on life and death;
2. incur potentially enormous expenses that fall to families, the government, or third party payers; and
3. (less nobly, but also significantly) justify expensive medical technology and research.

Confidentiality, Privacy, and Release of Information

Another way in which the constitutional right to privacy interacts with health care practice is through the legal protection of medical information. Information obtained from a patient through interviews, diagnostic tests, and treatments is all afforded protection under state law on confidentiality. This means that health care providers and institutions are prohibited from releasing medical information about a patient or former patient unless they receive a signed written consent by that person to release information, specifying what is to be released and to whom.

Many states have passed stringent laws and regulations specific to protect privacy around HIV testing status, and AIDS. For example, even if the patient gives general consent to release his/her medical record, the HIV test and related information must be deleted unless specifically requested by the patient. These stringent provisions are backed up by civil, and sometimes criminal, penalties for breaching the confidentiality required around a person's HIV status.

Health care workers may be informed in the course of rendering care, if that information is necessary to provide proper care and treatment. However, casual or unnecessary sharing of HIV information among coworkers or others not involved in the patient's care is unjustified invasion of privacy, and illegal in most jurisdictions. While many would argue that those who come in contact with a person infected with HIV have a right to know, the prevailing view is that proper practice involves the use of universal precautions with all patients. Beliefs about an individual's HIV status, therefore, are not determinative of whether the health care worker is placed at risk through giving care. By contrast, the potential damage done to an HIV-infected person through disclosing his/her condition can be devastating; psychologically, emotionally, economically, and socially.

Health care workers often lose sensitivity to the highly personal nature of the work they do. That insensitivity frequently manifests itself in casual conversations among co-workers, and even among friends outside the work place. Professionalism calls for retaining respect for and awareness of our patients' privacy. The law calls for careful observance of confidentiality in knowing and handling medical and health care information about others.

False Imprisonment

Although the term "false imprisonment" may sound quaint and unlikely in the context of delivery of health care, this is not the case. Nurses and physicians need to be acquainted with the principles, and ever respectful of the voluntariness, of submitting to health care required by American law.

A person is liable to another for the tort of false imprisonment if (s)he intentionally confines the other against his will within boundaries (s)he sets, and this confinement is maintained while the person confined is either conscious of the confinement or harmed by it. The implications of this abound in psychiatric-mental health treatment, pediatric, and residential care settings, but are not limited to these health care scenes.

The following case illustrates the point. An elderly gentleman was taken in by his son for admission to a nursing home. For the subsequent 3½ weeks following the gentleman's admission, he requested his own clothing from the nurses, and kept saying he wanted to go home, and that he did not want to be where he was. The nurses courteously and repetitively assured him that they understood he wanted to be home, but that he would "adjust" to his new surroundings. They told him that it was routine for new admissions to be in pajamas until they had been fully evaluated by the treatment team, and their care plan established. Requests by the man to make a phone call were answered with explanations of nursing home procedure disallowing money held by patients, and telephone use.

Convinced after 3 weeks of this that no one would take his wishes or communications seriously, the man found a ground level window that he was able to open and climb through. The indignity of escaping, clad in pajamas, and catching a city bus to seek help from a friend, was more tolerable than continuing imprisonment in the nursing home. He then hired a lawyer, brought suit against the nursing home for false imprisonment, and won.

Nurses are the front line of institutional health care. It is very often nursing judgment that determines which patient communications require responses, and what sorts of responses are appropriate. Be careful not to unwittingly patronize, or exploit the powerlessness of patients, by not listening to what they say.

AREAS OF EXPOSURE FOR NURSES

As discussed above, nurses are often treated under the law as agents of their employers with respect to liability for their acts. Known traditionally in the law as a "master-servant" relationship, this treatment can make the nurse personally liable, and make the nurse's employer legally liable. That relationship requires the nurse to use affirmative measures on behalf of patients to protect them from errors and omissions, or general incompetence, on the part of other health care providers. This obligation, according to both the courts and state departments of health, includes monitoring the physician, even if it means confrontation, to assure safe practice.

As nursing practice evolves to a role of increased independence, however, individual responsibility and liability also evolve and attach to that independence. In all situations of nursing practice, the nurse will be held to the standard of what a reasonably prudent nurse would do under the same or similar circumstances. If the setting is one in which specialized training is required for nurses to work, the nurse will be held to the standard of a reasonably prudent nurse with that specialized training. Accordingly, negligence may be found for varying levels of judgment or performance, based on practice settings of varying levels of specialized knowledge and skills.

An examination of the spectrum of nursing malpractice cases reveals five broad categories in which exposure to liability is customarily greatest for nursing professionals. These include the following:

Foreign Objects Left in Patients

Malpractice litigation frequently results from foreign objects being left in patients during surgical procedures. A study once conducted by the U.S. Department of Health and Human Services showed that 25 percent of alleged malpractice claims resulted from surgical material inadvertently being left in patients' bodies.

As a general rule, negligence is presumed to have occurred in instances where there has been a failure to remove a sponge or other device following a surgical procedure. The nurse who conducts an inaccurate instrument count is likely to be held liable jointly with the surgeon for negligence.

Improper Use of Equipment

Misuse of equipment such as mechanical monitors, defibrillators, resuscitation devices, infusion pumps, various measuring devices, and life-support systems represents another primary source of negligence claims. The hospital has a legal duty to exercise reasonable care in maintaining its equipment; the nurse has a legal duty to refrain from the unsafe use of potentially dangerous equipment. Nurses are responsible for routinely checking equipment to assure its readiness for use. Nurses also must know how to operate medical equipment safely and appropriately, and the equipment must be monitored while in use.

Improper Exercise of Physical Nursing Skills

This category comprises a number of common situations in which a nurse may fail to exercise reasonable professional skills. These situations include the following:

Leaving the patient unattended;
Failure to conduct a required examination;
Use of contaminated instruments;
Improper removal of catheters;
Improper administration of blood;
Misuse of hypodermic needles;
Failure to communicate with other members of the treatment staff;
Failure to make proper inquiries in preparing the patient's history; and
Failure to provide the physician with vital information regarding the
    patient.

When a nurse is working in conjunction with a physician, the physician often orders a specific medication in a certain dosage. If the patient is injured because the nurse fails to administer the correct medication in the correctly prescribed dosage, the nurse is likely to be held liable under a theory of negligence. Medications research has indicated that one medication error occurs for every seven or eight medications administered. This amounts to a 15 percent error rate. When projected on a national scale, this percentage suggests that of 10 million medications administered each day in the United States, 1½ million are administered in error. Understandably, medication errors constitute a large percentage of the medical malpractice cases brought under a negligence theory.

Failure to Observe and Report Symptoms

A large percentage of medical malpractice claims are rooted in communication breakdowns between nurses and physicians. Although nurses have no duty to diagnose the cause of a patient's ailment, they nevertheless remain legally obligated to report all of a patient's relevant symptoms to the physician in a careful and accurate manner. Although a heart-attack patient's symptoms may be readily observable, a nurse's responsibility is not to diagnose their cause, but rather to recognize their seriousness and report them to a physician as quickly as possible. Nonserious symptoms need not be reported immediately, but must always be recorded in the patient's chart to ensure that physicians and other medical personnel acquire knowledge of them.

Failure to Follow Physicians' Orders

The law requires nurses to make every best effort to follow physicians' orders. However, this law does not apply in instances where the nurse clearly recognizes that the patient will be injured if the physician's order is carried out. In the absence of such recognition, the nurse will normally remain immune from liability, provided he or she executes the physician's order in an appropriate professional manner.

LEGAL SIGNIFICANCE OF THE MEDICAL RECORD

Historically, the hospital's record regarding the patient was considered to be the hospital's property, including the nurse's notes. However, the courts in nearly all jurisdictions now accept the position that although the hospital may maintain custody of the records, those records are for the benefit of the patient, and are accessible to the patient. Most jurisdictions required that on the written request of the patient, or patient's representative, the hospital must release and deliver copies of all medical records and x-rays pertaining to that patient to his or her designated representative, or designated physician or hospital.

In light of the fact that the medical record of the patient is potentially subject to critical scrutiny by the patient, his or her authorized representative, governmental agencies, and the court system, the notations placed in that particular record are significant.

The nurse should keep in mind that medical records frequently serve as legal documents that may be introduced into court to prove that the care provided by the nurse and/or hospital representative or by a physician, breached acceptable standards of practice. An attorney for an injured party will use poorly written medical records to try to demonstrate that the nurse failed to follow the physician's order and failed to provide adequate care. Furthermore, the attorney will try and establish that the nurse's oral testimony cannot be believed because the care the nurse claimed he or she gave the patient was not charted. The attorney will try to establish that good nursing care dictates that significant observations be charted, and that if not charted, the care was in fact not given.

An attorney representing an injured party may attempt to prove the nurse's negligence by introducing copies of published standards while simultaneously pointing to the medical record errors and the omissions that suggest the standards where breached. Regardless of how good the nurse's performance actually may have been, the nurse's care may be found to be deficient simply because it was not documented in the patient's record.

Simply speaking, information contained in the chart is presumed to be true, and any activity omitted in charting is presumed not to have taken place. Additionally, many times the records are called into question many years after the care and treatment was given, when the nurse has no recollection of the patient, or the actual care and treatment. Accordingly, the records are extremely important in order to refresh the recollection of the nurse.

Retention of medical records is mandated by state and federal governments. The Joint Commission on Accreditation of Healthcare Organizations (JCAHO), supplies the following guidelines concerning medical records:

1. The Hospital maintains medical records that are documented accurately and in a timely manner, and are readily accessible, and permit prompt retrieval of information, including statistical information. The required characteristics are:

An adequate medical record is maintained for each individual who is evaluated or treated as an inpatient, ambulatory care patient, or emergency patient.

Some of the purposes of medical records are as follows:

To furnish documentary evidence of the course of the patient's medical evaluation, treatment, and change in condition during the hospital stay;

To document communication between the practitioner responsible for the patient and any other health care professional who contributes to the patient's care.

To assist in protecting the legal interest of the patient, the hospital, and the practitioner responsible for the patient.

2. The medical record contains sufficient information to identify the patient, support the diagnosis, justify the treatment, and

document the results accurately. The required characteristics are that the nursing notes and entries by non-physicians contain pertinent, meaningful, observations and information.

3. Medical records are confidential, secure, current, authenticated, legible, and complete. The required characteristic is that the hospital is responsible for safeguarding both the record and its informational content against loss, defacement, and tampering and from use by unauthorized individuals.

4. Individualized, goal-directed nursing care is provided to patients through the use of the nursing process. The required characteristics are:

Documentation of nursing care is pertinent and concise and reflects patient status.

Nursing documentation addresses the patient's needs, problems, capabilities, and limitations.

Nursing intervention and patient response are noted.

The importance of adequate, factual nursing documentation is obvious. The medical record contains nursing information that is essential not only to other health care professionals, but to researchers, as well as any other third party who can have access to the records. Nurses should be sure to document all the information that is necessary to communicate the patient's progress, all interventions taken, and all patient responses.

The medical record is not only a tool to document patient care, communicate, and educate, but it can also provide a legal defense in malpractice cases. The medical record serves the following functions:

1. Assist in planning patient care and in continuing the evaluation of the patient's condition and ongoing treatment;
2. Document the course of the patient's medical evaluation, treatment, and change in condition;
3. Document communication between the practitioner responsible for the patient and any other health professionals who contribute to the patient's care;
4. Assist in protecting the legal interests of the patient, the hospital, the practitioner responsible for the patient; and
5. Provide data for use in continuing education and research.

GOVERNMENTAL REGULATION OF NURSING PRACTICE

The practice of nursing in the United States has traditionally been regulated by the individual states. Each state gradually adopted laws that licensed nurses without attempting to regulate their professional conduct. Governmental agencies are now taking a much stronger role in regulating professional activities. Consequently nurses, as professionals, can find themselves being charged with unprofessional conduct by state licensing agencies. These charges can result in a variety of sanctions, including fines, and, in the most serious cases, license revocation. Nurses need to be aware of the state agencies that deal with licensing and the regulation of nursing practice because a professional disciplinary proceeding by a state agency can have serious consequences.

Those governmental agencies that nurses should be particularly concerned about are those that deal with federal and state drug enforcement. These agencies are concerned with administration, dispensing, and prescribing of controlled substances.

Many states have laws and regulations that define professional misconduct, and can apply to nursing practice. Among the actions that are considered professional misconduct are the following:

1. Obtaining a license fraudulently;
2. Fraudulent practice, including practice beyond its authorized scope;
3. Being habitually substance-impaired and/or practicing one's profession while substance-impaired or under a physical or mental disability;
4. Permitting practice by an unlicensed person; and
5. Committing unprofessional conduct.

Actions constituting unprofessional conduct include the following:

1. Gross negligence;
2. Filing a false report required by law or by the Education Department;
3. Divulging confidential information without a patient's consent;
4. Delegating professional responsibilities to a person who is not qualified to perform them; and
5. Performing professional services which have not been authorized by the patient.

Unprofessional conduct specific to health professions, including nursing practice, includes the following:

1. Abandoning or neglecting a patient in need of immediate care;
2. Failure to maintain an accurate medical record reflecting the evaluation and treatment of each patient; and
3. Failure to use scientifically accepted infection prevention techniques.

The foregoing are offered here to illustrate the conduct for which a nurse can be sanctioned by the state. Penalties can range from having one's professional license placed on probationary status, through permanent revocation and fines.

MALPRACTICE PREVENTION AND PRECAUTION

Actual malpractice, in which there has been an error or omission on the part of the nurse causing injury to the patient, does occur and will continue to occur. Nursing in this day and age is complex. Nurses are sometimes placed in unique and uncomfortable positions in many employment settings, particularly in hospitals, clinics, and health maintenance organizations. The nurse is not only required to follow orders given that deal with the patient's care and management, but is also required to use independent nursing judgment in assessing a patient and reporting symptoms and observations.

Often, it is the nurse who spends the most time with the patient, and the nurse is required to perform all of his or her functions in an orderly, knowledgeable way in a very demanding setting. These demands subject a nurse to a risk of malpractice litigation resulting from any perception on the part of the patient that something untoward happened.

Medical malpractice exists because human beings make errors, and nurses are going to make errors. However, there are many situations where malpractice has not, in fact, been committed, and where there is no genuine basis for a medical malpractice lawsuit, but where the patient still retains counsel to go forward with litigation. Conversely, there are also many situations where actual malpractice has taken place, and yet no suit is instituted against the hospital, doctor or nurse. Sometimes this is because the patient is unaware that a breach of duty caused him or her "injury." Other times, patients understand that a mishap has occurred, yet there continues to exist a satisfactory health care provider/patient relationship.

For a patient to reach the point where he or she actually consults with an attorney, and thereafter formally retains an attorney to bring a malpractice suit, it is commonly the case that the patient has become angry with the health care provider, and that that provider has not taken appropriate actions to diffuse the anger. This is a common underlying cause for a patient to seek satisfaction through the legal system. In effect, the physician or nurse has not been successful in maintaining rapport with the patient, the patient's expectations are not being met, and the patient has lost confidence in the physician, nurse, or hospital.

Although no list of do's and don'ts will prevent a malpractice claim against a nurse, the nurse who is conscientious and practices according to the following principles decreases the probability of becoming a defendant:

1. Be an active practicing nurse who keeps abreast of his or her particular specialty area by being active in professional societies. Subscribe to and read journals in your specialty, follow the literature, and participate in continuing education programs.

2. Keep abreast of changes in statutes, rules, regulations, and legal decisions that affect your legal responsibilities to the patient.

3. Learn how to operate specific equipment that you will be using in care and treatment of your patients. Be aware of the safety features on the equipment that you are using, and of the safety steps that are to be taken before the equipment is utilized.

4. Document appropriately, accurately, and legibly, and under no circumstances make any alterations on the record, subsequent to an incident or a registered complaint. Be knowledgeable in the hospital's policies and procedures, and follow these policies and procedures. Additionally, the nurse should be knowledgeable with regard to standards published by JCAHO and the American Nurses Association. The nurse will be presumed to know the hospital's policies and procedures, and also presumed to know the pertinent standards of JCAHO and the American Nurses Association; failure to follow these could serve as a basis for a finding of negligence.

5. Make sure that the "right hand knows what the left hand is doing." It is important for the nurse to remember that (s)he is part of a treatment team that involves other nurses, technical people, and physicians. A lack of communication between health care professionals resulting in injury to the patient could serve as a basis for a negligence claim.

6. The nurse should be familiar with package inserts on the drugs that are prescribed and ordered. If a reasonably prudent nurse would not have administered the medication ordered, because it was improper, or the dosage was improper, then there could be a finding of negligence on the part of the nurse for having carried out the particular order.

7. The nurse should know his or her own physical limitations as well as professional limitations. The nurse should not be undertaking procedures for which (s)he is not fully qualified, and/or for which (s)he has not been trained.

8. Demonstrate and show that you have empathy and that you are a caring individual. You will diminish the probability of being named as a defendant in a lawsuit when your patients believe that you are concerned about their well-being.

TOPICS FOR DISCUSSION

1. What are the four conditions which must be met if an individual is to be found liable?

2. Are nurses legally responsible for obtaining the consent of the patient for surgery? Explain the nurse's role in this procedure.
3. Are nurses legally responsible for reporting changes in the patient's condition to the physician?
4. What precautions should nurses observe to protect the patients' rights of privacy?
5. Will the legal liability of nurses increase as their role expands?
6. List the eight steps outlined by the authors to decrease the probability of nurses being involved in malpractice claims.
7. If you were in charge of a nursing home and a very elderly and confused patient decided he wanted to leave the home (against the physician's advice) what laws would you consider? How would you handle the situation?

REFERENCE

Douthwaite, G. (1987). *Jury instructions on medical issues*, third edition (pp. 340–341). Charlottesville, VA: The Michie Company.

5

Nursing Theory: History and Critique

Bonnie Bullough

Theories are formal statements that are constructed in order to organize ideas and explain events. People feel more comfortable if they can explain why certain events reoccur. Even the ancient peoples had theories as to why the sun came up each morning, or why the seasons changed. Their theories helped them predict what would happen next, so they could know when it was time to plant and when it was time to store foods for the impending winter. Our current explanations for those events may be more sophisticated, but that does not negate the usefulness of those earlier theories at the time they were constructed.

As nursing becomes more scientific, theory is becoming a more important part of our knowledge base. The profession has moved beyond a body of knowledge which can be passed on from one generation of nurses to another in an apprenticeship format, or a set of procedures, to a more formalized body of knowledge including empirically tested theories. Theory is actually a shorthand way of storing research findings. It summarizes empirical research and allows for further testing as well as use of the findings in the practice setting. A more formal definition of theory which is often cited is the one written by Kerlinger (1973):

> A theory is a set of interrelated constructs (concepts) definitions,
> and propositions that present a systematic view of phenomena
> by specifying relationships between variables, with the purpose
> of explaining and predicting the phenomena. (p. 9)

This definition restricts theory to those statements which specify the relationships between the concepts (or variables) in order to predict phenomena. Once a prediction is made it can be tested, so this definition restricts the term "theory" to theories which can be tested using a scientific methodology.

Nursing has, however, developed one group of theories which are not particularly testable. These are the grand theories of nursing. Consequently, a less demanding definition of theory may be more useful for understanding the full range of extant nursing theory. The definition proposed by Barnum (1990) would include the full range of theories in nursing:

> A Theory is a statement that purports to account for or characterize some phenomenon. (1989, p. 1)

There are a variety of systems for classifying theories. The system presented here uses five levels, ranging from the most simple to the most complex. Only the first three levels are testable so they are the only theories which would fit the Kerlinger definition. However, since the last two levels use the word "theory", all five levels need to be understood. These five levels are listed and explained below.

FIVE LEVELS OF THEORY

1. Descriptive theory
2. Correlational theory
3. Explanatory theory
4. Grand theory
5. Meta theory

A *descriptive theory* defines or describes something. Sometimes a descriptive theory merely names a concept; asserting, for example, that there is such a thing as self-concept. At a more complex level, the descriptive theory may describe a process, as do the various developmental or staging theories. For example, Kubler-Ross described the stages people go through in the grieving process, starting with a denial of the loss and ending up with full acceptance (1969). The developmental theories of Erickson and Piaget, which concern the processes children go through in growing up, are descriptive theories.

A *correlational theory* relates two variables but does not indicate which variable causes the other. Correlational theories are not very common because they tend to be a transitional phase in the theory development process. Researchers who want to develop explanatory theories may first test the fact that two variables relate to each other before trying to show that one of the variables is causal to the other. An example of this type of theory development can be seen in an article by Jacqueline Sherman and her colleagues. They are studying factors related to obesity in preschool children including the mother's knowledge of nutrition, her ideas about ideal infant body size, her ethnicity, and, if she is Mexican-American, her level of acculturation to American norms (Sherman, Alexander, Clark, Dean, & Welter, 1992). Eventually some or all of these variables might be used in an explanatory theory. In the case of Sherman et al., it is clear that this is not yet an explanatory theory because the causal direction of some of the variables is not yet established. For example, a high ideal body weight might cause the mother to overfeed her child, but on the other hand, having an obese child might cause the mother to change her ideas as to what the ideal body size should be.

An *explanatory theory* explains why certain concepts are clustered. One example is the Health Belief Model, which was developed in the early 1960s by a group of social psychologists who wanted to predict the decisionmaking process involved in seeking preventive health services such as immunizations. They based the theory on the phenomenological work of Kurt Lewin, who held that it is the world of the perceiver that determines action rather than just the objective facts (Becker, 1974; Rosenstock, 1974). The Health Belief model holds that people will take preventive action if (1) they believe that a certain illness will negatively alter their lives, (2) they are susceptible to the illness, and (3) the benefits of taking the preventive action will outweigh the barriers or costs to taking the action. The process can also be influenced by cues to action, such as public education campaigns or advice by health care providers. These cues bring the problem of the disease to the minds of the subjects so that they consider the three variables in the model. Nurses have used the Health Belief model to predict which women will practice breast self-examination (Massey, 1986), and to understand decisions about estrogen replacement therapy (Logothetis, 1991). Use of the Health Belief model by nurses and other researchers concerning condom use as a preventive measure for Autoimmune Deficiency Syndrome (AIDS) indicates that most heterosexual Americans are mistakenly convinced that they are not particularly susceptible to the disease, so the use of condoms or other barrier contraceptives is dangerously low (Becker & Joseph, 1988; Bridgers, Figler, Vaughn, & Sawin, 1990).

Grand theory attempts to explain a whole system, or a very broad range of events. It is often so large and complex that it cannot be tested. Some theory analysts call these "conceptual" models to differentiate them from testable theories, but the term grand "theory" will be used here. Grand theory in nursing was very important in the 1970s as nurses, including Calista Roy (1976), Dorothy Johnson (1959, 1961, 1974) and Martha Rogers (1970) sought to advance the profession by defining nursing so as to differentiate it from medicine (Torres, 1986). These can also be thought of as prescriptive theories, since their originators argued that nurses should conceptualize their work using the concepts outlined in the theory.

Selected grand theorists of nursing will be discussed in this chapter, a somewhat longer list is presented in Table 5.1.

Meta-theories are clusters of theories which are used to analyze the differences and similarities in a group of theories. Meta-theorists such as Meleis (1986) and Flaskerud and Holleran (1980) have analyzed the grand theories of nursing to identify the themes which run through them, and to show how they are similar or different.

Formatting Theories

Certain conventions are followed in the structuring of theories. Ordinarily, the essence of the theory is presented in the form of a declarative sentence which is called a *proposition*. This proposition is made up of one or more *concepts,* so sometimes theories are called *conceptual frameworks.* If the theory is *descriptive,* the major proposition will merely indicate that a certain phenomenon exists and that a concept is defined in a certain way. If the theory is *correlational* or *explanatory,* it will explain how two or more variables fit together.

Since theories are made up of concepts, it is important to understand what a concept is. A *concept* is a word or a cluster of words describing an object, idea or event. It is the mental image of the phenomenon rather than the actual physical thing. Concepts can be either concrete, which means that they are basic, like the color "blue", or they can be more complex, such as " blue sky."

Concepts can be nonvariable or variable. When a concept simply labels an item, such as a chair, it is nonvariable; the mental image evoked by the word is the only form of the phenomenon. When the concept has more than one form it is variable. For example the concept "anxious" varies, with some people being more anxious than others. Fawcett and Downs (1986) use the examples of the concept "nursing care" to explain a

TABLE 5.1 Grand Nursing Theories

Date	Theorist	Theory
1966	Hall	Caring (defined as teaching)
1967	Levine	Four Conservation Principles
1970	Rogers	The Science of Unitary Human Beings
1971	Orem	Self-care deficit
1971	King	Interacting systems framework
1972	Neuman	Health Care systems model
1974	Roy	Adaptation model
1976	Johnson & Aiger	Behavioral systems
1976	Paterson & Zderad	Humanistic nursing
1979	Watson	Caring
1981	Parse	Man-Living-health

nonvariable concept; but the term "quality of nursing care" is variable, because it can be measured on a scale from high quality nursing care to low quality.

Concepts are often clustered by researchers to form ideas about the variables they want to study. These concepts are called *constructs;* for example, the construct of "self-esteem" or "gender dysphoria." Constructs are used by researchers to better explain and measure the phenomena of interest. They include more than one idea, but the ideas are clustered to form the constructs. The researcher who invents or popularizes a particular construct will often develop a scale to measure it.

The theory may also include assumptions which are statements about the phenomenon. While these are not tested, they form a backdrop for thinking about the major concepts and how they are related to each other. It is important to understand the assumptions of the theory. For example, a nursing theory that assumes that all people want to recover could be erroneous in its assumptions if there are actually people who are ready to die.

Theory Construction

Theories can be constructed using two different processes. The most common approach is to draw generalizations from research findings or empirical observations. This is called the *inductive* approach to theory-building. The theory can then be used to guide further research, which in turn tests the theory and determines whether or not the generalization holds true over time.

The second method of theory construction is *deductive*, sometimes called the "armchair approach." Using a philosophical belief as a starting point, some people use a *deductive* approach by working the theory out in their head, and then testing it with empirical observations at a later time. Some theorists leave the task of testing the theory to other people.

THE HISTORICAL DEVELOPMENT OF THEORY IN NURSING

Nurses started developing an interest in theory in about 1960. There were by that time a growing number of nurses with baccalaureate education and a few who held graduate degrees, providing a nucleus of nurses with the educational background necessary to understand the concept of theory. A review of the literature of that era suggests that the primary motivation for developing a theoretical basis for nursing practice seems to have been a desire on the part of nurses for the status of a profession. For example, in the *American Journal of Nursing,* Genevieve and Roy Bixler (1959) analyzed the status of nursing as a profession and found need for change, including the development of a specialized body of knowledge; education in colleges instead of hospital training schools; and more autonomy in the patient care decisionmaking process. On the other hand, nursing was clearly professional in its dedication to provide much needed service to the public. Using medicine and law as the models, other writers of this period reiterated the position that nursing and the other "semi-professions", such as social work and librarianship, would need to increase their bodies of theoretical knowledge in order to be considered professions (Barber, 1963; Goode, 1966; Greenwood, 1957).

The Yale Theorists

The earliest concentrated focus on theory in nursing developed at Yale. Two philosophers, James Dickoff and Patricia James, worked with Ernestine Wiedenbach, an emeritus professor of maternal and newborn nursing, to outline a process for developing theory in a practice discipline. They published a series of papers in *Nursing Research* arguing that theories of a practice discipline should provide the bridge between practice and research, and that theoretically based research was the key to broadening nursing knowledge. Their work did much to shape the subsequent development of theory in nursing (Dickoff, James, & Weidenback, 1968). Even the terms they used appear in some of the later grand theories of nursing. For example, they used the term "agency" to describe the nurse or the health care provider, and the term "patiency" to describe the client or patient. These concepts can be noted in Orem's theory of self-care (1985).

Theorizing at Yale continued under a group of social scientists who were hired as faculty members in the school of nursing. Their focus was on the social and psychological aspects of illness and health care. Powhaton Wooldridge worked with graduate nursing students to develop what he called practice theory. These were a group of hypotheses which were tested to identify useful approaches to lessening the stress of illness and treatment. As the hypotheses were tested, they were clustered to form practice theory about nursing interventions which lessened stress (Wooldridge, 1983).

The Grand Theories of Nursing:
Dorothy Johnson and the University of California
at Los Angeles Group

Contemporary with the Yale theorists were a group of grand theorists of nursing who defined nursing in broad outlines. They tended to be concentrated in certain centers, with the University of California at Los Angeles (UCLA) and New York University (NYU) furnishing the leadership to the movement. Dorothy Johnson, a UCLA faculty member, started working on a theoretical framework for nursing in the 1950s. Her most important contribution was probably not her grand theory, which was published later, but her definition of nursing as focusing on the caring elements of patient management, in distinction to the physician's role, which was said to be the treatment of illness.

Johnson's first paper on this topic, published in 1959, outlined her philosophy of nursing, arguing that the key element was hands-on nursing services. She defined these services as *caring for*, rather than *curing* the patient (Johnson, 1959). Her thinking in this regard was influenced by Frances Kreuter (1957), who argued that the health care delivery system should be changed to develop specialized nurse clinicians who would be paid more money, yet be allowed to remain at the bedside instead of having to move up the administrative hierarchy in order to advance in the field. Kreuter described the role of the clinician as specializing in care:

> Care is expressed in tending to another, being with him, assisting, protecting . . . providing for his needs and wants with compassion—tenderness. (Kreuter, 1977, p. 140)

Johnson was also influenced by the sociologists who were her contemporaries. She often referred to a paper by Miriam Johnson and H. W. Martin (1958) which used a structural functional theoretical approach to analyze the role of nurses. These authors argued that nurses maintained the social system of the doctor-nurse-patient triad by managing the equilibrium within the system and creating a therapeutic environment. Whenever the physician's treatment plan seemed harsh or was unclear to the patient, the nurse would explain and clarify it so that it could be tolerated. She would restore a calm atmosphere if the patient were distressed, and care for the emotional needs of the physician and other workers so that a therapeutic environment could be maintained (Johnson & Martin, 1958).

Florence Nightingale's writings were also a part of the discussion. Though Nightingale (1860) saw nurses as subservient to physicians, she also believed nursing might possibly be more important than medicine because feeding patients and managing their environment could often keep them alive while nature cured them. Johnson's definition of caring was more similar to Nightingale's approach than to the more tender, empathetic aspects of nursing mentioned by Kreuter. The definition of caring Johnson used defined caring as basic nursing procedures: comfort measures, environmental management, emotional support, and teaching. She believed that physicians could be as kind as nurses, but that they focused their work on curing, rather than sustaining, the patient (1959, 1961, 1974).

This emphasis on caring was broadly accepted, and Johnson's dichotomy between caring and curing became a common element in the grand theories of nursing which followed (Rogers, 1970; Roy, 1976, 1984). The emphasis on nursing care defined as social psychological support, teaching, and sustaining care was termed the "professional role" by the American Nurses Association (ANA) in its 1965 position paper *Educational Preparation for Nurse Practitioners and Assistants to Nurses*. The term "nurse practitioners" referred to baccalaureate-educated nurses, differentiated from "technical nurses", who were focused on curing the patient and serving physicians (ANA, 1965). This same position was reiterated in the ANA *Social Policy Statement* (1980).

Johnson herself eventually developed a grand theory which focused on behavioral systems as alternatives to the traditional physiological systems. Descriptions of this theory were published in 1976 by Aiger and in 1980 by Johnson. Other UCLA students and faculty members, Calista Roy and Betty Neuman, constructed major grand theories, while conbutions to the analysis of nursing theory were made by Afaf Meleis, Joanne Rheil, and Cynthia Scalzi.

Roy's Adaptation Model

The most well-known of the California theorists was Sister Calista Roy, a student of Dorothy Johnson's, who was also a teacher of nursing at Mount Saint Mary's College in the Los Angeles. The major focus of Roy's theory is on behavioral science concepts, with the individual described as a participant in bio-psycho-social adaptive systems. Patients are described as being under varying degrees of stress, and their goal is to adapt to that stress.

Roy identifies four adaptive modes which are used in this circumstance. The role of the nurse in this system is to identify the stress in the patient's life; classify the adaptive mode being used, and help patients adapt to stress by manipulating the environment. The nurse can be conceptualized as an external regulatory force. Roy defines adaptation as the individual's ability to cope with the constantly changing environment. The Roy Adaptation model has been adopted by many schools to guide their curricula. In addition, in the 1980s, several Canadian hospitals moved to adopt the model to structure nursing practice.

Betty Neuman: Health Care Systems

The Neuman systems model is drawn directly from general systems theory, so it uses all of the terms of that model. Systems theory, a mid-twentieth century theory used in a variety of disciplines, focuses on interrelationships between the subsystems (or parts of the system). Outcomes are influenced by factors that are inside or outside the system. Systems models often use squares or circles to illustrate how the system works, showing the input to the system, the processes within the system, the output from the system, and how feedback to the system can occur (Dultd & Giffin, 1985).

The Neuman model pictures patients as being at the center of the system, where they are influenced by physiological, psychological, social, and environmental variables. Nurses can improve the health and welfare of patients by manipulating the variables which impact upon them. The systems format allows the theory to be very broad in scope, so it has proven to be very useful as a structure for curriculum development in schools of nursing (Neuman, 1982).

Martha Rogers: The Science of Unitary Human Beings

The theory devised by Martha Rogers, former Chair of the Department of Nursing at NYU, has had a significant following in nursing. The principles of Rogers' theory are said to be drawn from the laws of homeodynamics, although the theoretical or research base in physics or any other recognized discipline is not clear. The theory was originally called a "unitary theory of man", but it was changed to "unitary human beings" to fit current nonsexist language norms. First published in her 1970 book, *An Introduction to the Theoretical Basis of Nursing*, Rogers' theory conceptualizes people as involved in dynamic energy fields which are contiguous with energy fields outside of their bodies. The major propositions of the theory explain the principles of reciprocity between these energy fields, as well as synchrony and helicy (Rogers, 1970).

This theory has changed over time as many graduates of the NYU program have worked to shape it with their dissertations and other research (Moody & Hutchinson, 1989). Rogers herself also continues to work on and revise the theory. One of her recent speeches focused on its applications to an understanding of aliens in outer space (Rogers, 1990).

The most well-known implementation of the theory was devised by Dolores Krieger, who designed a treatment modality using therapeutic touch. In a 1975 article published in the *American Journal of Nursing* she reported increased hemoglobin levels among a sample of patients who had been treated with therapeutic touch. A 1979 book amplified her technique. Krieger defines health as a harmonious exchange between the individual's energy fields and those in the surrounding environment. A lack of harmony causes pain or illness. Krieger claimed that therapists could internalize the disordered energy and restore it to balance, so patient's bodies can heal themselves (Krieger, 1975, 1979).

Studies of the method by followers of Kreiger were able to demonstrate relaxation related to therapeutic touch (Heidt, 1981; Quinn, 1984). However, as the research became more rigorous and controls for placebo effects were included, it became clear that although touch can have an anxiety-relieving function, there is probably no scientific basis for believing that people can be cured of anything by a therapist who claims to channel their energy fields with his or her hands (Clark & Clark, 1984; Keller & Bzdek, 1986; Sandroff, 1980).

In spite of this, Paul T. Hageman, who earned his doctorate in nursing at New York University, established a federally funded clinic in Buffalo, New York, to treat people using therapeutic touch. He and the therapists he trains were described as using a focused intent to channel life energy, helping their patients to release blockages and bring their energy fields into harmony and balance (When healing requires, 1992).

Another follower of Rogers, Rosemarie Rizzo Parse, has combined the Rogerian science of unitary human beings with the traditional philosophy of existentialism, calling the theory a Man-Living-Health system (1981).

Dorothea Orem's Self-Care Deficit Theory

The grand theory proposed by Dorothea Orem has been widely used to guide both nursing practice and curriculum. It was originally designed as a framework for a practical nursing curriculum and later extended to the professional level of nursing. A basic assumption of the theory is that people who are well carry out the various activities of daily living themselves. Illness is defined by this model as a state in which the individual is incapable of maintaining those self-care activities. This deficit can be taken over by others including nurses. Nursing care is therefore defined as filling these deficits.

Orem's framework for the nursing role is a traditional role, but its emphasis on self-care has been appreciated as the consumer movement has developed and people have spoken out in favor of having more power over their own health care (Orem, 1971, 1985).

Imogene King's Interacting Systems Framework

Imogene King proposed another general systems theory involving the four major domains of nursing: people, environment, nursing, and health. The nurse-patient interaction is implemented in an interpersonal system. Effective interaction patterns are a tool of good nursing care (King, 1981). The King theory is probably the most testable of the grand theories of nursing, because hypotheses can be generated about the interaction patterns.

Jean Watson's Science of Human Caring

The most recent of the grand nursing theorists is Jean Watson, who defines the nursing role as caring for people. While she accepts the traditional grand theory definition of caring as what nurses do that is aside from what physicians do, she adds several other components, including an existential or spiritual dimension. The relationship is a mutual one between the nurse and patient, which includes the following ten factors:

1. Humanistic-altruistic system of values
2. Faith-hope
3. Sensitivity to self and others
4. Helping-trusting, human care relationship
5. Expressing positive and negative features
6. Creative problem-solving caring process
7. Transpersonal teaching-learning
8. Supportive, protective, and/or corrective mental, physical, societal and spiritual environment
9. Human needs assistance
10. Existential-phenomenological-spiritual forces

(Watson, 1985).

Functions of Theory in Nursing

Four major phenomena were identified by the grand theorists of nursing as the domain of interest to the profession: patients (or persons), nursing, the environment, and the health-illness continuum (Fawcett, 1984; Flaskerud & Halloran, 1980). Staking out this claim was, in fact, a major function of the grand theories. These theorists never argued that members of other disciplines could not practice or do research in these domains, but that nursing should and could.

In order to understand the need for this positive assertion of territoriality, it is necessary to understand the subordinate position held by nurses in the past, particularly in relationship to physicians. This relationship was well illustrated by the early state medical practice acts which were written into law in the nineteenth century before any other health care occupations had practice acts. These acts described physicians as the persons who were responsible for all health care. This meant that when the other practice acts were written, in the twentieth century, they had to carve out a piece of medicine's territory (Bullough, 1980). This was relatively easy for dentistry and veterinary medicine, because their independence did not impinge on medicine; but nursing, podiatry, pharmacy, and physical and occupational therapy are still involved in the process of negotiating their boundaries vis-á-vis the more expansive medical practice acts. The grand nursing theories can be thought of as one mechanism employed by the profession to claim its place in the sun. The grand theorists of nursing were however, very modest in their claim to territory, limiting their focus only to the "caring" aspects of patient management, and repeatedly pointing out that the kind of nursing they espoused did not overlap with the physician's mission to cure.

Another function of the grand theories was to structure nursing curricula. The standards for accreditation of baccalaureate and higher degree nursing programs enunciated by the National League for Nursing in the 1970s indicated that there should be an appropriate use of theory to guide the curriculum. Most schools interpreted this to mean that the school should adopt one grand theory to use with all patient populations. The very broad theories such as the ones constructed by Neuman, Roy and Orem, lent themselves well to this use. Since the theory structured the students' learning of the nursing process, the tenets of the theory carried over into their practice settings.

As the criteria for accreditation evolved in the 1980s, schools moved on to use more testable theories that are limited in scope, that is, child development theories in pediatric courses, theories of stress in the critical care courses, and so on, so the grand theories are less important now as curriculum devices and in practice settings, although some Canadian hospitals are now moving to structure nursing practice using the grand nursing theories.

A major failure of the grand theories was that they were not very useful in the scientific enterprise. They were seldom used in the research process and when they were used it was to identify a phenomenon of interest to the researcher, rather than to construct testable hypotheses from the propositions of the theory (Silva, 1986). This suggests that the grand theories of nursing may not be theories at all, but rather *philosophies* of nursing. Calling them philosophies may make their functions seem more congruent with reality.

Consequently, the major focus of published nursing research is now on testable theories which describe concepts of concern to nurses, or describe the relationship between two or more variables to illuminate a patient care situation. Using the format outlined in this chapter, these theories are at the descriptive, correlational, or explanatory levels. Some writers call these theories of the middle range. At first these are theories were drawn directly from the behavioral sciences, but over time nurses became less shy about constructing, adapting, and synthesizing middle-range theories to fit the patient care situation. As a result there are now several major testable theories which can reasonably be called nursing theories. Good examples of these theories are those developed by Pender (1982) to predict preventive health behaviors, the Wallston theory of health locus of control (Wallston, Wallston, Kaplan, & Maides, 1976), Leininger's identification of the cultural aspects of caring (1970, 1977), and Benner's (1984) work identifying the difference between the practice of novice and experienced nurses.

Issues Related to The Life Cycle of Theories

This historical description of the theories in nursing has indicated that they have changed over time. This raises the question as to whether a change in the theoretical underpinnings of a profession is legitimate or inconsistent. This author argues that not only is change legitimate, but that probably all theories have a finite term of usefulness. Even before nurses themselves started theorizing, the theories which they adopted changed as the theories of society changed. For example, when the accepted childrearing practices were rigid or even punitive, nurses supported these ideas; nurses taught mothers to use rigid feeding schedules, and that sparing the rod would spoil the child. As the ideas of Freud and others refocused childrearing practices to make them more permissive and supportive, nurses relaxed their own approach.

The fact that theories can have a useful life span and then be overturned is an important point made by the philosopher of science, Thomas Kuhn (1970), in his book on the structure of scientific revolutions. He reviewed the ancient geocentric theory which held that the universe circled around the world, and noted that eventually findings made by navigators and astronomers cast doubt on its validity. It had, however, become entrenched in people's minds and even in religious beliefs, so the change to a heliocentric theory was not easy. Kuhn argues that the old theory was useful and helped to make sense of the world, but the change, which he calls a scientific revolution or a shift in paradigm, was necessary.

One example of a theory from the health field which served for a time and was then overturned is the theory of miasma. *Miasma* was defined as a form of bad air, or bad odor, that permeated places where rotting organic material was located. Florence Nightingale accepted the theory of miasma and believed it caused illness, but did not accept the germ theory which held that there were microorganisms which caused disease. She advocated scrubbing the sickroom and getting rid of everything that looked dirty or smelled bad, and consequently the practices she advocated helped to prevent disease.

The belief in miasma as the basis for infectious diseases was also held by Edwin Chadwick, a lawyer and secretary of England's Poor Law Commission, who was influential in bringing about public health reforms in nineteenth-century England. Chadwick used the theory of miasma to explain the high death rate among London's poor and argued that the problem could be remedied by getting rid of the open sewers and the rotting garbage that covered the streets. Eventually his ideas on sanitation were adopted and the death rate in London fell (Bullough & Rosen, 1992). In the last part of the nineteenth century, miasma theory was overturned by the findings of Koch and Pasteur, making it clear that pathogenic microorganisms were the cause of diseases that had been attributed to miasma. Their findings were so important that this is sometimes called the bacteriological revolution. Nevertheless, the theory of the disease potential of miasma was very useful during its lifetime, even though it was eventually overturned and corrected by an improved theoretical formulation.

Issues Related to the Primacy of Care

The dichotomy between the elements of care and cure posited by the grand theorists of nursing has served as a significant barrier to the development of the nursing specialties that overlap with medicine. As indicated in Chapter 1, the nursing specialties started moving into the master's-level framework after 1965, when the federal government started granting funds for graduate nursing education. Although nurse educators of that era tended to be enthusiastic about the development of the clinical specialist role, many of them questioned the validity of the nurse practitioner role. These educators conceptualized the role of the nurse as sharply different from that of the physician, which was described as curative. Because the CNS role was focused on meeting the psychosocial needs of patients, teaching, and consultation, it was considered legitimate, but the mixed role of the NP, which drew from both medicine and nursing was considered illegitimate. Martha Rogers, who was probably the most colorful of the critics of the NP role, perceived its development to be a ploy to lead nurses away from their rightful place and into the orbit of medicine. She argued that NPs had in effect left the nursing profession and they should be forced to drop the name "nurse" (Rogers, 1972). Nurse educators who accepted this line of thinking were naturally unwilling to accept NP programs into their schools. This lack of acceptance was a barrier to the early institutionalization of NP education into the mainstream of nursing education. This same belief system made other programs which overlapped with medicine—nurse anesthesia, nurse midwifery, and critical care nursing—equally unwelcome in most nursing graduate programs during the 1970s and even into the 1980s. The concentration of the nursing theory enterprise at New York University also served as a barrier to the legal acceptance of those nursing specialties which overlapped with medicine, because the theorists and their followers were able to get the care–cure dichotomy written in the New York State Nurse Practice Act in 1972. This legal recognition moved the focus of the diagnostic process away from the patient to the worker, and separated the nursing diagnosis and treatment plan from a medical one. "Diagnosis" as defined in New York as follows

> [Diagnosis] in the context of nursing practice means the identification of and discrimination between physical and psychosocial signs and symptoms essential to the effective execution and management of a nursing regime. Such diagnostic privilege is distant from a medical diagnosis. (New York State Education Law, 1972)

This wording was immediately adopted in 13 other states, and several other states added the concept of a nursing diagnosis and/or a nursing regime to their laws (Bullough, 1980). This significantly popularized the nursing diagnostic taxonomies, which focused nursing concern away from the patient's curative needs and emphasized needs for emotional support and teaching. Counsel to the Board of Regents in New York indicated in 1974 that this language put the nurse practitioner role outside the law. Consequently, their practice was significantly curtailed until the nurse practitioners were able to get the practice act amended in 1989 to make their full practice legal (New York State Education Law, 1989).

Thus the influence of the grand theorists of nursing was significant in separating the advanced specialties which developed after 1965 into two distinct models: the Clinical Nurse Specialist and the Collaborative model of nursing which overlaps with medicine. The nursing specialties which fall under this second model include nurse practitioners, nurse anesthetists, nurse midwives, and the critical care nurses. Nurses who specialize in psychiatric/mental health nursing may also fit into this model because they treat patients. These specialists are moving away from their totally care-oriented colleagues to joined the list of treatment-oriented professions which includes medicine, osteopathy, dentistry, clinical psychology, and podiatry. Figure 5.1 shows these two models.

Thus the development of the grand theories of nursing, with their heavy emphasis on the caring orientation, has had a profound influence on nursing, with both positive and negative consequences. These theories certainly emphasized the importance of patient teaching and emotional support as components of the nursing role, but the desire to separate

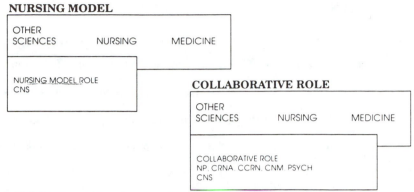

NURSING MODEL

OTHER
SCIENCES   NURSING   MEDICINE

NURSING MODEL ROLE
CNS

COLLABORATIVE ROLE

OTHER
SCIENCES   NURSING   MEDICINE

COLLABORATIVE ROLE
NP, CRNA, CCRN, CNM, PSYCH
CNS

* All candidates have a basic nursing degree first.

FIGURE 5.1 Alternative educational models for advanced specialty practice *Nursing and Health Care.* (1992). Bonnie Bullough, Alternative models for Specialty Nursing Practice. *Nursing & Health Care, 13,* 257.

nursing from the curative elements of patient care has made the development of the advanced collaborative specialties more difficult.

SUMMARY

This chapter has presented the concept of theory and identified the development of theory in nursing, particularly since 1960. Early theorizing focused on the grand theories of nursing, which were for the most part not testable. They did, however, popularize a philosophy of nursing which avoided the curative elements of health care and emphasized the caring elements. The researchers in nursing have now moved on to an emphasis on theories of the middle range, which are testable.

TOPICS FOR DISCUSSION

1. Should nurses focus their role on caring and leave the curing of illness to physicians?
2. Why should theories be tested?
3. Have the grand theories helped nursing to advance?
4. Have the grand theories been a deterrent to nursing's development of its body of knowledge?
5. Was the theory of miasma as a cause of disease a useful theory, even though it did not hold up over time?

REFERENCES

Aiger, J. (1976). *Behavioral Systems and Nursing.* Englewood Cliffs, NJ: Prentice-Hall.

American Nurses Association. (1965). *Educational preparation for nurse practitioners and assistants to nurses.* Kansas City, MO: Author.

American Nurses Association. (1980). *A social policy statement.* Kansas City, MO: Author.

Barber, B. (1963) Some problems in the sociology of professions. *Daedalus, 9,* 669–688.

Barnum, B. J. S. (1989). *Nursing theory: Analysis, application, evaluation* (3rd ed.) Glenview, IL: Scott Foresman/Little, Brown.

Becker, M., & Joseph, J. (1988). AIDS and behavioral change to reduce risk: A review. *American Journal of Public Health, 78,* 394–410.

Becker, M. H., Kaback, M. M., & Rosenstock, I. M. (1975). Some influences on public participation of genetic screening programs. *Journal of Community Health, 1,* 3–14.

Benner, P. (1984). *From novice to expert: Excellence and power in clinical nursing practice.* Menlo Park, CA: Addison-Wesley.

Bixler, G. K., & Bixler, R. W. (1959). The professional status of nursing. *American Journal of Nursing, 59,* 1142–1147.

Bridgers, C., Figler, K., Vaughn, S. & Sawin, K. (1990). AIDS belief in young women: Are they related to AIDS risk-reduction behavior? *Journal of the American Academy of Nurse Practitioners, 2,* 107–112.

Bullough, B. (Ed.) (1980). *The law and the expanding nursing role.* New York: Appleton-Century-Crofts.

Bullough, B., & Rosen, G. (1992). *Preventive medicine in the United States from 1900 to 1990.* Nantucket, MA.

Bullough, V. L. (1980). Licensure and the medical monopoly. In B. Bullough (Ed.), *The law and the expanding nursing role* (pp. 14–22). New York: Appleton-Century-Crofts.

Clark, P. E., & Clark, M. J. (1984). Therapeutic touch: Is there a scientific basis for the practice? *Nursing Research, 33,* 37–41.

Creasia, J. L., & Parker, B. (1991). *Conceptual foundations of nursing practice.* St. Louis, MO: Mosby-Year Book.

Dickoff, J., James, P., & Wiedenback, P. (1968). Theory in a practice discipline: Part I. *Nursing Research, 17,* 415–435.

Dickoff, J., James, P., & Wiedenback, P. (1968). Theory in a practice discipline: Part II. *Nursing Research, 17,* 545–554.

Duldt, B. W., & Giffin, K. (1985). *Theoretical perspectives for nursing.* Boston: Little, Brown.

Erickson, E. (1963). *Childhood and society.* New York: Norton.

Fawcett, J. (1984). *Analysis and evaluation of conceptual models in nursing.* Philadelphia: Davis.

Fawcett, J., & Downs, F. (1992). *The relationship of theory and research* (2d ed.). Philadelphia: Davis.

Flaskerud, J. H., & Holloran, E. J. (1980). Areas of agreement in nursing theory development. *Advances in Nursing Science, 3,* 1–7.

Goode, W. (1966). Librarianship. In H. M. Vollmer & D. L. Mills (Eds.), *Professionalization* (pp. 34–43). Englewood Cliffs, NJ: Prentice-Hall.

Greenwood, E. (1957). Attributes of a profession. *Social Work,* 2, 45–55.

Heidt, P. (1981). Effect of therapeutic touch: An anxiety level of hospitalized patients. *Nursing Research, 30,* 32–37.

Johnson, D. (1959). A philosophy of nursing. (1959). *Nursing Outlook, 7,* 198–200.

Johnson, D. (1961). The significance of nursing care. *American Journal of Nursing, 61,* 63–66.

Johnson, D. (1974). Development of a theory: A requisite for nursing as a primary health profession. *Nursing Research, 23,* 372–377.

Johnson, D. E. (1980). The behavioral system model for nursing. In J. P. Rheil and C. Roy, (Eds.), *Conceptual models for nursing practice* (pp. 207–216).

Johnson, M. M., & Martin, H. W. (1958). A sociological analysis of the nurse role. *American Journal of Nursing, 58,* 374–377.

Keller, E., & Bzdek, V. M. (1986). Effects of therapeutic touch on tension headache pain. *Nursing Research* 35, 101–106.

Kerlinger, F. N. (1973). *Foundations of behavioral research* (2nd ed.) New York: Holt, Rinehart and Winston.

King, I. (1971). *Toward a theory for nursing.* New York: Wiley.

King, I. (1981). *Toward a theory for nursing.* New York: Wiley.

King, I. (1981). *A theory for nursing: Systems, concepts, process.* New York: Wiley.

Krieger, D. (1975). Therapeutic touch. The Imprimatur of nursing. *American Journal of Nursing, 75,* 784–789.

Krieger, D. (1979). *Therapeutic Touch: How to use your hands to help or heal.* Englewood Cliffs, NJ: Prentice Hall.

Kreuter, F. R. (1957). What is good nursing care? *Nursing Outlook, 5,* 302–305.

Kübler-Ross, E. (1966). *On Death and Dying.* New York: Macmillan

Kuhn, T. S. (1970). *The structure of scientific revolutions* (2nd ed.). Chicago: University of Chicago Press.

Leininger, M. (1970). *Nursing and anthropology: Two worlds to blend.* New York: Wiley.

Leininger, M. (1977). The phenomenon of caring: Part V. caring: the essence and central focus in nursing. *Nursing Research Report, 2,* 2–14.

Levine, M. E. (1967). The four conservation principles of nursing. *Nursing Forum, 6,* 45–59.

Logothetis, M. L. (1991). Women's decisions about estrogen replacement therapy. *Western Journal of Nursing Research, 13,* 458–474.

Massey, V. (1986). Perceived susceptibility to breast cancer and practice of breast self-examination. *Nursing Research, 35,* 183–185.

Meleis, A. (1985). *Theoretical nursing: Development and progress.* Philadelphia: Lippincott.

Meleis, A. I. (1986). Theory development and domain concepts. In P. Moccia (Ed.), *New approaches to theory development* (pp. 3–21). New York: National League for Nursing.

Moody, L. E., & Hutchinson, S. A. (1989). Relating your study to a theoretical context. In H. S. Wilson (Ed.), *Research in nursing* (pp. 275–332). Menlo Park, CA: Addison-Wesley.

Neuman, B. M., & Young, R. J. (1972). A model for teaching a total person approach to patient problems. *Nursing Research, 21,* 264–269.

Neuman, B. (1982). *The Neuman systems model.* Norwalk, CT: Appleton-Lange.

New York State Education Law. (1972). Op Title 8, Article 139 Chapter 6901.

New York State Education Law. (1989). Op Title 8, Article 139, Chapter 6901, 6910.

Nightingale, F. (1946). *Notes on nursing.* Philadelphia: Lippincott (original work published 1860).

Orem, D. M. (1985). *Nursing concepts of practice* (3rd ed.). New York: McGraw Hill.

Parse R. R. (1981). *Man-living-health: A theory of nursing.* New York: John Wiley.

Paterson, J. G., & Zderak, L. T. (1976). *Humanistic nursing.* New York: Wiley.

Pender, N. L. (1982). *Health promotion in nursing practice.* Norwalk, CT: Appleton-Century-Crofts.

Piaget, J. (1958). *The growth of logical thinking from childhood to adolescence.* New York: Basic Books.

Quinn, J. F. (1984). Therapeutic touch an energy exchange: Testing the theory. *Advances in Nursing Science. 6,* 42–49.

Rogers, M. E. (1970). *An introduction to the theoretical basis of nursing.* Philadelphia: Davis.

Rogers, M. (1972). Nursing: To be or not to be. *Nursing Outlook, 20,* 42–46.

Rogers, M. (Sept. 30, 1990). Keynote Address, Nursing Theory Association of Community Health Nursing Educators, American Public Health Association Meeting, September 30, 1990. New York.

Rosenstock, I. M. (1974). Historical origins of the health belief model. In Becker, M. H. (Ed.). *The Health Belief Model and personal health behavior* (pp. 1–8). Thorofare, NJ: Charles B Slack.

Roy, C. (1983). *Introduction to nursing: An adaptation model* (2nd ed), Englewood Cliffs, NJ: Prentice-Hall.

Sandroff, R. (1980). A skeptic's guide to therapeutic touch. *RN, 43,* 25–30, 82–83.

Sherman, J. B, Alexander, M. A., Clark, L., Dean, A., & Welter, L. (1992). Instruments measuring maternal factors in obese preschool children. *Western Journal of Nursing Research, 14,* 555–575.

Silva, M. (1986). Research testing nursing theory: State of the art. *Advances in Nursing Science, 96,* 1–11.

Torres, G. (1986). *Theoretical foundations of nursing.* Norwalk, CT: Appleton-Century-Crofts.

Wallston, K. S., Wallston, K. A., Kaplan, G. D., & Maides, S. A. (1976). Development and validation of the health locus of control scale. *Journal of Consulting and Clinical Psychology, 44,* 580–585.

Walker, L. O., & Avant, K. C. (1988). *Strategies for theory construction* (2nd ed.) Norwalk, CT: Appleton & Lange.

Watson, J. (1979). *The philosophy and science of caring.* Boston: Little, Brown.

Watson, J. (1985). *Nursing: Human science and human care: A theory of nursing.* Norwalk, CT: Appleton-Century-Crofts.

When healing requires the right touch, D'Youville students are taught laying-on of hands as therapeutic treatment. (1992, March 10). *Buffalo News,* p. C3.

Wooldridge, P. J., Schmitt, M. H., Skipper, J. K., & Leonard, R. C. (1983). *Behavioral science and nursing theory.* St. Louis: Mosby.

PART II

Selected Clinical Issues

6

Nurse-Midwifery Today

Lisa Monagle

The profession of midwifery has ancient origins, and today, despite past and present obstacles, the practice of nurse-midwifery in the United States is stronger than ever. Never before have so many professional positions been left unfilled at ever-increasing salary levels. Educational opportunities for potential nurse-midwives have also expanded, both in terms of the number of schools offering programs and the structure of the programs being offered, allowing more home study and flexibility for the potential student. In this chapter, definitions of practicing midwives, including international midwives, certified nurse-midwives, and professional and lay midwives, will be given. Thereafter, the history of the profession of nurse-midwifery in the United States will be presented, followed by a description of the educational programs currently in place. The nurse-midwifery scope of practice will then be outlined and the latest legislative update summarized. Finally, the current barriers to the long-term and expanding practice of nurse-midwifery in the United States will be discussed.

DEFINITIONS OF PRACTICING MIDWIVES

On an international scale, midwifery is a recognized and highly regarded profession with practitioners found throughout the world. The International Congress of Midwives generally defines a midwife as a graduate of a fully recognized midwifery educational program in the country in which the midwife is located who has acquired the requisite qualifications to be registered and/or legally licensed to practice midwifery. The international sphere of practice includes the necessary supervision and care of women from pregnancy, labor and the postpartum period, to care for the newborn and infant, as well as adding the important component of counseling and education, not only for patients, but also within the family and community. It is estimated that 80% of the world's babies are delivered by midwives. This, combined with the profession's emphasis on preventative health care, represents a major contribution of midwifery to the health of women and children worldwide.

According to the American College of Nurse Midwives (ACNM) (Directory of Nurse-Midwifery Practice, 1992), a certified nurse-midwife (CNM) is an individual educated in the two disciplines of nursing and midwifery, who possesses evidence of certification according to the requirements of the American College of Nurse-Midwives. Traditionally, the potential certified nurse-midwife has entered a master's level or post-baccalaureate certificate program after having completed a four-year baccalaureate of science in nursing. In addition to certication by the ACNM, state requirements for the practice of nurse-midwifery, which vary from state to state, must also be met. Upon successful completion of the certificate or master's level nurse-midwifery program and the ACNM board exam, certified nurse-midwives then undergo registration according to the regulations for the state in which they have chosen to practice.

In 1992 the American College of Nurse Midwifery issued the following definition:

Nurse-Midwifery practice is the independent management of women's health care, focusing particularly on pregnancy, childbirth, the postpartum period, care of the newborn, and the family planning and gynecological needs of well women. The Certified Nurse-Midwife practices within a health care system that provides for consultation, collaborative management or referral as indicated by the health status of the client. Certified Nurse-Midwives practice in accord with the *Standards for the Practice of Nurse-Midwifery*, as defined by the American College of Nurse-Midwives, (1992). Nurse-midwifery practice includes services for healthy women and their babies in the areas of prenatal care, labor and delivery management, postpartum care, normal newborn care, family planning, and well woman gynecology.

In the United States, non-nurse-midwives have also been practicing the art of midwifery. Non-nurse-midwives include lay midwives, whose training is not standardized, and trained professional midwives, whose training is standardized and approved by state regulating boards, under whose regulations professional midwives practice. As of 1992, while all 50 states regulate the practice of CNMs, 26 states also regulate the practice of midwifery performed by midwives who are not certified nurse-midwives (Barickman, Bidgood-Wilson, & Ackley, 1992). While the numbers of practicing *non*-nurse-midwives are believed to be relatively small, this "sister" profession represents two decades of challenge to the consideration of nursing as the essential basis for further midwifery education. The controversy is ongoing, and has resulted in significant legislative changes regarding midwifery practice most recently in the state of New York, these will be further discussed in the nurse-midwifery legislation section.

HISTORY OF NURSE-MIDWIFERY IN THE UNITED STATES

For centuries, obstetrics, defined by many dictionaries as the practice of the art of midwifery, was the sole province of the midwife. Initially, in colonial America, much honor was afforded the original midwives, and their importance to other segments of the population through the years has been well documented. Despite their initially honored status, however, a series of factors reduced midwifery from a status of respect to one of disrepute by the early 1900s. These factors included the replacement of midwives by the developing practice of physicians, as well as socioeconomic factors such as the influx of immigrants, inadequate education, and the lack of organization among the practicing midwives.

In the early 1900s, a debate over what was known as "the midwife problem" took place. From 1912 to 1914, medical schools began to include obstetrics in their curricula, and obstetrics became an established medical specialty by 1930. The obstetrical branch of the medical profession had grown in influence, and they strongly opposed midwives on grounds that their practice inhibited the growth and advancement of obstetrics as a recognized medical specialty, and that the midwives lacked standardized training. Obstetric care began a mass movement out of the home into the hospital, and laws were passed to regulate the practice of the indigenous midwives. By 1940, the majority of births were recorded in hospital settings and were attended by physicians.

Second, a public health campaign against disease, malnutrition, dirt, and uncleanliness was growing. Because the midwife was largely associated with the lower socioeconomic classes—typically being a member of the immigrant group she would serve—she and her work were seen as substandard and unclean. Finally, a major concern surrounding the high mortality rates developed in the 1920s among public health officials. Again, because of the midwives' involvement in the care of women from lower socioeconomic classes, combined with their lack of standardized training and professional organization, the midwife was seen as being associated in part with poor pregnancy outcomes.

By the early 1970s, 97% of all births were attended by physicians (Institute of Medicine, 1982). The move toward hospital birth had occurred quickly in the 1930s, but because of the lack of standardized obstetric training among the physicians themselves, their high use of obstetrical instruments and interventionist approaches and the continued lack of access by the poor to medical care, maternal and infant mortality rates remained high. Public Health officials suggested that implementing a standardized training program for nurse-midwives might fill the gap in access to medical care and contribute to the care of the uncomplicated obstetric patient. This suggestion was not supported by the medical profession until after the Frontier Nursing Service nurse-midwives demonstrated excellent outcomes and the Maternity Center Association, a training program for nurse-midwives, was opened in the 1930s.

The birth of American nurse-midwifery occurred in 1925, when Mary Breckenridge, an American nurse educated in nurse-midwifery in England, began the Frontier Nursing Service, which served one of the poorest and most isolated areas of Kentucky. In its first 7 years, one thousand mothers and their infants were cared for, and maternal and infant mortality in the area was reduced dramatically. In 1931, the Maternity Center Association opened the country's second nurse-midwifery service, caring for immigrants living in New York City's West Side. The Maternity Center was seen as a major force in the significant improvements in the health of mother and babies in New York at that time (Tom, 1982). In 1955, the American College of Nurse-Midwives was formed to represent the needs and concerns of nurse-midwives and to accredit educational programs, and since then the growth of nurse-midwifery in the United States has been slow but steady.

In the 1970s, new interest has widely developed in the psychological factors surrounding the birth experience. The changing social contexts in which contemporary childbirth interests are expressed include the women's movement, consumerism, the desire for more natural deliveries, and concern about rising health care costs. The effect of this new consumer interest has been a re-examination of obstetrical practices and the increased involvement of nurse-midwives, lay midwives, family medical physicians, and other health care practitioners in the care of the childbearing family.

NURSE-MIDWIFERY EDUCATIONAL PROGRAMS

Currently, there are 37 programs to educate nurse-midwives that are accredited or pre-accredited by the ACNM Division of Accreditation and the U.S. Department of Education (Whitfill & Burst, 1993). These include 11 certificate (or 18-month) programs, 25 master's degree (or 24-month) programs and 1 pre-certification (or new) program (Directory of Nurse-Midwifery Practices, 1992).

Nurse-midwifery students typically begin their midwifery training with extensive prior experience in maternity and public health nursing. A student nurse-midwife then receives intensive instruction (often with a ratio of 1:1) in clinical midwifery and advanced training in normal obstetrics, gynecology, and newborn care.

In a continuing attempt by the ACNM to expand the numbers and vary the structures of nurse-midwifery programs, the Community Based Nurse-Midwifery Education Program (CNEP) was pre-accredited in 1987 with the idea of offering didactic and clinical learning opportunities to nurse-midwife students in their own community setting. Currently, 320 students are enrolled in the CNEP program, attending 2 week sessions per year at the administrative headquarters in Kentucky, and corresponding with program coordinators regarding didactic and clinical progress. Thus far, the major obstacle to the acceptance of nurse-midwifery students to this new program has been a lack of clinical practice sites within easy access to the potential student. Overall, however, the CNEP educational program has singlehandedly been responsible for a striking increase in nurse-midwifery student enrollment.

NURSE-MIDWIFERY'S SCOPE OF PRACTICE

Today, there are over 4,500 certified nurse-midwives in the United States. Furthermore, the ACNM has launched a new educational objective of promoting strategies to reach the number of 10,000 nurse-midwives practicing by the year 2000. Currently, nurse-midwives are working in a wide variety of settings: hospitals, birthing centers, health maintenance organizations, public health departments, private practices, and clinics. Although nurse-midwifery started in this country as a service available only to the poor and disadvantaged, nurse-midwives now serve women from all economic classes and practice in all settings where American women choose to give birth. The majority of nurse-midwives continue to deliver babies in hospitals or birthing centers attached to the hospitals. A small percentage of nurse-midwives, however, also attend home births, whose numbers are now estimated to be about 1% of the total number of births per year.

The practice of nurse-midwifery has recently been closely tied to the concept of and practice involvement in birth centers or nonhome, out of hospital delivery centers. The number of birth centers have also grown from 3 in 1975 to 153 in 1992 (Directory of Nurse-Midwifery Practices, 1992). Birth centers and home deliveries constitute an alternative health movement which has developed to promote practices associated with individual choice in the activity of the laboring woman, such as a home-like atmosphere for the birth, and family participation and control in the birth. This development occured as an opposing force to conventional obstetrics, which has tended to emphasize procedures to deal with group risks, such as infection, monitoring fetal and neonatal well-being, and a hospital atmosphere with nearness to equipment and use of technology.

In the practice of nurse-midwifery in birth centers and home deliveries, the primary controversy surrounds safety issues. While physicians, nurse-midwives, and midwives each hold strong opinions on the relative safety of hospital, birthing center, and home births, large-scale research remains unavailable to conclusively determine risk assessments for the three birthing sites. Data collection is ongoing to compare the outcomes of home and birthing center births to hospital deliveries for women with similar risk factors.

In any setting, however, the provision for the safety of mother and baby has always been a primary concern of the nurse-midwife. Over the years, nurse-midwives have maintained a superb record of safety and client satisfaction. Research shows that a women experiencing a healthy pregnancy, labor, and delivery is as safe in the hands of a nurse-midwife as she would be in the hands of a physician. A report by the Institute of Medicine (1982) emphasized that nurse-midwives are particularly effective in managing the care of pregnant women, and that such care results in fewer premature and underweight babies, indicating a significant level of professional recognition on the part of the physicians.

NURSE-MIDWIFERY LEGISLATION

Certified nurse-midwives are professionally recognized in all 50 states. Laws governing the practice of midwifery and the nature of the regulating boards, however, vary from state to state. Currently, nurse-midwifery is regulated by a Board of Nursing in 34 states and the District of Columbia, Virgin Islands, and Puerto Rico. Four states have set up a joint regulation of nurse-midwifery by their Boards of Nursing and Medicine. Four states are currently regulated by their Department of Public Health. In three states, nurse-midwifery is regulated by only their Board of Medicine. Two states are regulated by a Committee of Certified Nurse-Midwifery, and one state falls under a mixed statutory authority.

On June 25, 1992, new legislation for New York State midwives was signed into law. It was specifically designed to recognize the profession of midwifery as separate from either medicine or nursing, the new legislation represents a significant new direction by recognizing the practice of non-nurse midwifery professionals. The full implications of the new legislation and formal break with nursing as a requisite base to the practice of midwifery in the state of New York remain to be more fully understood with time.

Regarding prescription-writing priviledges, 36 states including the District of Columbia grant the authority for writing prescriptions to Certified Nurse-Midwives. Moreover, 27 state jurisdictions mandate private insurance reimbursement for Nurse-Midwifery services. 26 state jurisdictions regulate the functioning of birth centers.

Finally, with regard to professional reimbursement issues, nurse-midwifery services are routinely covered by many major insurance groups. Most private medical insurance carriers as well as the Civilian Health and Medical Program of the Uniformed Services (CHAMPUS), Medicaid and Medicare recognize the quality of care and reimburse all standard services performed by the nurse-midwives.

BARRIERS TO NURSE-MIDWIFERY PRACTICE

While most nurse-midwives would acknowledge the professional practice as exciting and deeply rewarding, a number of difficult barriers to nurse-midwifery practice remain. One of the strongest obstacles to current and future practice is the insufficient number of certified nurse-midwives from which to recruit for many available positions. Hundreds of nurse-midwifery positions are available nationally which remain unfilled for long periods of time. The lack of numbers of practicing nurse-midwives in turn restricts the ability to educate nurse-midwifery students through preceptorships and adds to the frustration of nurse-midwives waiting to expand their practice settings or obtain scheduling relief through the hiring of new professional colleagues.

A second barrier to the successful long-term practice of nurse-midwifery remains that of burn-out. Long office hours, combined with a frequent call schedule, make the nurse-midwifery profession physically demanding. The long hours are then frequently combined with the on-going need for each nurse-midwife to lobby local legislators, to remain politically "on alert," and to engage in public relations efforts to explain the practice of midwifery to the public and other health care professionals on an ongoing basis. These demands are difficult to fulfill after a number of years in practice.

A third obstacle to a rewarding nurse-midwifery practice is the philosophical differences in practice between the nurse-midwives and one or more of their physician partners in practice or physician consultants. The lack of suitable physician collaboration results in more stressful working conditions. In some cases the nurse-midwife may need to compromise her philosophical beliefs about the way in which obstetrics should be practice in order to gain the ability to practice with the essential physician backup; or wait for practice opportunities with other physicians whose philosophy of practice may be more congruent with that of the nurse-midwive's. Furthermore, despite the existence of formal physician backup or consultation documents, some nurse-midwives experience ongoing discomfort and uncertainty, regarding how supportive partners or consultants will be in varying circumstances, including potential lawsuits.

A fourth obstacle to nurse-midwifery practice remains the difficulty in finding the physician backup so crucial to the successful practice of nurse-midwifery in rural or home birth practices. While nurse-midwifery is widely accepted among practicing physicians, the low number of rural physicians and the lack of desire on the part of physicians to be involved with home births results in difficulties in establishing either rural or home birth nurse-midwifery practices.

A fifth obstacle is the presently resolved but constantly threatening problem of the availability of malpractice insurance. The lack of affordable malpractice insurance for obstetricians, and, by association, nurse-midwives, reached a crisis level between 1984 and 1986, spurred by the number of obstetrics-related claims which tripled in the previous six years. Although the outcomes of nurse-midwives practice were well documented as not contributing to this increased law suit risk, some insurance companies decided suddenly to discontinue the coverage of nurse-midwives. This resulted in a number of nurse-midwifery practices closing, with a resultant number of nurse-midwives temporarily out of work. Given the wide publicization of this crisis period, the career of the nurse-midwife was frequently characterized as a high-responsibility, high-risk, and relatively low-paid profession, an impression which may have lingered among and turned away many potential students.

A final obstacle to the growing practice of nurse-midwifery in the United States is the lack of previous business and/or administrative experience of the nurse-midwives. In addition to the burden of the long hours described above, some nurse-midwives find themselves, because of the ever-evolving nature and shortages characteristic of the profession, in positions of administration or business development. This can be an additional stress for those who feel ill-prepared for other nonpractice-related professional involvement.

Despite all these obstacles and barriers to the growing, long-term, rewarding practice of nurse-midwifery, the profession remains strong and ever growing. Many professional opportunities of all types abound, and salary ranges are higher than ever, with clinical positions typically being advertised for nurse-midwives in the $50,000 to $60,000 range for assignments in the larger cities. The profession of nurse-midwifery is now solidly respected by all groups, including medical colleagues, government officials and the lay public.

SUMMARY

The practice of midwifery, or "being with women" is a profession as old as the beginning of time. It is a profession which is ever evolving, growing in the United States and world wide. Despite the current shortages of trained nurse-midwives and the obstacles to practice presently experienced, the future looks brighter than ever for this rewarding and dynamic profession.

TOPICS FOR DISCUSSION

1. Is nurse-midwifery practice currently legal in all 50 states?
2. Do nurse-midwives currently have prescription writing privileges in the 50 states?
3. What is the role of the physician in the successful nurse-midwifery practice?
4. What do present-day midwives and nurse-midwives have in common with their historical counterparts?
5. Does the profession of nurse-midwifery appear to have a future in the medical system?
6. Should out-of-hospital deliveries assisted by nurse-midwives, such as those occurring in birth centers or in homes, be encouraged or discouraged?
7. What are the implications of birth center or home deliveries for the cost to the medical system?
8. What are some pros and cons of the New York State legislative movement toward recognition of the profession of midwifery as separate from nursing and medicine?
9. What are some of the barriers to the current practice of nurse-midwives?
10. How can these barriers be effectively and realistically addressed in the promotion of one of the oldest professions, midwifery?
11. Internationally, what roles might be possible for the American trained nurse-midwife?

REFERENCES

American College of Nurse-Midwifery (July 27, 1992). *Position Statement: Definition of Nurse-Midwifery Practice*. Washington, D.C.
Barickman, C., Bidgood-Wilson, M., & Ackley, S. (1992). Nurse- midwifery today: A legislative update, Part II. *Journal of Nurse-Midwifery, 37*, 175–209.

Institute of Medicine, Division of Health Sciences Policy and National Research Council Commission on the Life Sciences. (1982). *Research issues in the assessment of birth settings: Report of a study by the committee on assessing alternative birth settings.* Washington, DC: National Academy Press.

Tom, S. (1982). Nurse-midwifery: a developing profession. *Law, Medicine and Health Care, 10,* 262–266.

Whitfill, K., & Burst, H. (1993). ACNM-accredited nurse-midwifery education programs: Program information. *Journal of Nurse-Midwifery, 38,* 216–227.

7

The Role of the Nurse as a Mandated Reporter of Child Abuse

Adele R. Pillitteri

A recent national survey has projected that nearly 1.5 million children and adolescents are subjected to abusive physical violence each year (Straus & Gelles, 1990). When instances of sexual and emotional abuse and neglect are added to this number, abuse of children may occur to as many as 23 of every 1000 children. It rates as one of the most frequently seen child health problems in the United States today.

HISTORICAL PERSPECTIVE

Parental harm of children is not a new social problem. The killing of children, or infanticide, was practiced in ancient civilizations. Biblical references such as the story of Moses (Exodus 1:22) describe the killing of all male infants. The Laws of the Twelve Tables in Rome not only condoned but encouraged the destruction of infants born with disabilities. Hospital records from the 1800s show preschoolers admitted with gonorrhea, long bone fractures or neglect, diagnoses that suggest child abuse (Pelletteri, 1993). During the Industrial Revolution, children as young as 5 were employed in the United States. Some of these children were chained to machines to keep them from running away (Lazoritz, 1990). Such treatment seemed justified because children were viewed as the property of their parents, and parents could therefore treat them in any way they chose.

Child abuse was first recognized as a social problem in the United States when in 1873, a nurse, Etta Wheeler, learned of a 7-year-old girl named Mary Ellen who was being kept as a prisoner in a dark, unventilated room and subjected to severe daily beatings. Ms. Wheeler appealed for help for Mary Ellen to police and child benevolent societies, but found them unable to help her, based on the premise that children were the property of their parents. As a last resort, Wheeler pleaded with Henry Bergh, the founder and president of the Society for the Prevention of Cruelty to Animals, for help. Bergh arranged to have Mary Ellen removed from her home. Due largely to the awareness raised by the publicity of this one child's plight, the following year, in 1874, the Society for the Prevention of Cruelty to Children was founded.

Child abuse became recognized as a medical problem in 1946 when Caffey (1946), a radiologist, reported the association of multiple bone fractures and subdural hematomas in children as possibly being caused by trauma. Sixteen years later, Kempe, Silverman, Steele, Droegmuller, and Silver (1962) coined the term "Battered Child." A hundred years after Mary Ellen needed to be rescued from a stepparent by a society to protect animals, the federal government passed a law to protect children from abuse: the Federal Child Abuse Prevention and Treatment Act of 1974. This act requires health care personnel to identify and report abuse in children (Lazoritz, 1992).

At the time this reporting law was passed, the average nurse worked in a hospital setting. The responsibility for the identification and reporting of child abuse, therefore, routinely passed up the rank to a physician, so although the issue concerned nurses, few were actually directly involved in filing a report on suspected abuse.

As nursing roles have become more extensive and autonomous with the 1980s and 1990s, the responsibility for identifying and reporting child abuse has increased or moved from a "never" to a "probable" nursing role. This increased responsibility raises issues that nurses have never before needed to consider.

DEFINING CHILD ABUSE

Section 3 of the Federal law, The Child Abuse Prevention and Treatment Act of 1974 (PL 93-247), defines child abuse as:

> the negligent treatment or maltreatment of a child under the age of 18 by a person who is responsible for the child's welfare under circumstances which indicate that the child's health and welfare is harmed or threatened thereby. . . .

Specific legal definitions of abuse are established in the United States at the state level, along with which persons in that state have been named as *mandated* reporters (persons who must report child abuse when they recognize it or pay a penalty for failure to do so) and *permissive* reporters (people who *may* report abuse but would not suffer a penalty if they failed to report).

Nurses are designated as mandatory reporters (those who must report) in all states, either by being directly named in the law, or referred to under the broad categories of "health care agency employee" or "practitioner of the healing arts." Some states maintain a narrow list of mandated reporters. Others, like California, designate a broad range including film processors. This category of people was included because of the possibility that they process and see child pornography films. A number of states (Indiana, Maryland, New Jersey, and Texas, for example) have such broad mandatory reporting laws that they designate *anyone who has reason to believe a child has been subjected to abuse* as a mandatory reporter.

An important component of all these state statutes is that the person filing the report does not have to *confirm* abuse; only *suspect* it. It means that neither the child or a parent has to admit that abuse occurred for a report to be filed. Abuse reporting laws are written with an *immunity* provision that guarantees the reporter can not be prosecuted for the report if the report later proves to be false as long as the report was made in "good faith." A consumer group, Victims of Child Abuse Laws (VOCAL), has been formed to aid parents who are wrongly accused of child abuse (Wong, 1987). The few law suits brought either independently or by this consumer group against mandated reporters has established the precedent that immunity is absolute; as long as the report was made in good faith, the reporter has no reason to fear retaliation for filing a report.

In the majority of states, the penalty for not reporting abuse is viewed as a misdemeanor and the penalty is a 6-month jail sentence plus a fine of between $500 and $1000. Maryland, in contrast, views the failure to report as a felony and sets the penalty as a 15-year jail sentence (Dobbs, 1986). In addition to these penalties, if a nurse failed to report suspected abuse and further injury occurred to a child, the nurse might be subject to malpractice action or loss of license.

In most hospitals today, a nurse suspecting that abuse may have occurred still may not actually file the official report; a member of the medical staff (perhaps an emergency room physician) or the chairperson of a child abuse treatment team is responsible for this. This system is organized to save time by limiting the number of reports coming from a single facility. The nurse does have a responsible role to alert the designated reporter of his or her suspicions that a child has been abused. This person would then examine the child, confirm the abuse, and file the report.

In many emergency departments, nurses work independently to obtain an admission or triage history. If such a nurse suspected abuse, but the parents left with the child before a physician could see the child, the nurse would have the responsibility to alert the designated reporter that abuse was suspected, and the report should then be filed on the nurse's suspicions alone. Nurses working in emergency rooms should reassure themselves by discussing the issue with the designated reporter of their facility and make certain that this procedure would be followed should the situation occur. Otherwise, they leave themselves open to failing to report.

California's law is hallmark legislation in this area, as it assures the autonomy of nurses by stating that "no supervisor or administrator may impede or inhibit the reporting duties (of child abuse) and no person making such a report shall be subject to any sanction for making the report" (CA Penal Code, Section 11166F).

In a setting where a nurse's judgement was not respected, or where she or he could not convince the designated agency abuse reporter to file a report, the nurse could file an anonymous report independently of the agency. This type of action is not preferred, however, because anonymous reports are not apt to provoke the same level of child care protection agency response as official reports, as only 13% of anonymous reports are found to be factual, whereas 42% of official reports are accurate (Schetky, 1986).

A number of nurses maintain such independent practices that they are directly responsible for reporting. A community or home care nurse who suspects abuse has occurred in a home setting, for example, has this full responsibility; so does a nurse practitioner or clinician who sees children independently.

In those states where they are not specifically designated as mandated reporters, nurses would be well advised to petition their state legislatures to have the category of registered nurse added to the list of mandated reporters. Although this increases nurses' responsibilities, it also empowers nurses in an instance where they believe that abuse has occurred (for example, a 6-month-old child seen in an emergency room for the fifth time in 4 months for "falls down the stairs" has the injuries discounted by a young housestaff physician as "boys will be boys"). Being listed as a mandatory reporter also makes an explanation to parents about why the report was filed easier "The law requires that I do this". It also better protects against a suit brought by the parents if the report should prove to be false (the nurse was specifically mandated to make the report).

Nurses need to be certain that they are well informed on the subject of child abuse and are capable of recognizing abuse so they do not over- or underreport it.

TYPES OF CHILD ABUSE

Child abuse can be divided into the five major categories shown below:

1. *Physical Abuse*: defined as the intentional, nonaccidental use of physical force or an intentional nonaccidental act of omission aimed at hurting, injuring or destroying a child (Gil, 1971).

    A. *Shaken Baby Syndrome*: a form of abuse in which an infant is shaken causing cerebral and retinal damage (Spaide, Swengel, & Mein, 1990).

2. *Emotional Abuse*: defined as the damage or impairment of a child's emotional condition. This may include verbal abuse (belittling, scapegoating, humiliation, or verbal threats).

    A. *Munchausen Syndrome by Proxy*: a form of child abuse in which a parent creates fictitious illness in the child by falsifying history or altering laboratory reports, subjecting the child to unnecessary medical procedures or hospitalization (Senner & Ott, 1989).

3. *Physical Neglect*: a large category that can be divided into a number of subdivisions.

    A. *Abandonment*: the expulsion from the home (temporary or permanent) or the chronic shuttling of a child among caretakers.

    B. *Inattention to Health Care*: delay or failure to seek care for an obvious illness, failure to allow reasonable diagnostic maneuvers, failure to follow through with reasonable, prescribed treatments, or failure to obtain immunizations.

    C. *Inadequate Supervision*: children left alone or with only a preteenage child as supervisor.

    D. *Avoidable Inattention to Hazards*: the failure to protect children from poisons, exposed wiring, and dangerous structural aspects of a home, such as open windows and staircases or exposure to frostbite or extreme sunburn.

    E. *Deprivation of Necessities*: failure to provide adequate food, clothing or shelter, or failure to attend to a child's personal hygiene to the point where the child becomes ill or infested.

    F. *Educational Neglect*: the failure to enroll a child in school, facilitate attendance or cooperate with educational plans, or failure to respond to chronic truancy.

    G. *Permitting or Condoning Maladaptive Behavior*: Permitting substance abuse, prostitution or delinquency.

4. *Emotional Neglect*: is the outright rejection or conspicuous absence of support or care about a child's emotional well-being.

5. *Sexual Abuse*: is the molestation or sexual injury of children that includes a broad category of offenses.

A. *Incest*: sexual intercourse with a close relative.

B. *Promoting Prostitution*: urging or encouraging a child to engage in prostitution.

C. *Pornography*: obscene photography, filming or depiction of children for commercial purposes or the arousal or gratification of either the perpetrator, child or viewing audience.

DETECTING CHILD ABUSE

Child abuse may be suspected at a number of different points in child–nurse health care contact.

History Taking

Parents should be able to account for any injury on their child's body, excluding an occasional ecchymotic mark that has occurred from bumping into an object or playing a contact sport.

When describing an injury that resulted from abuse, parents may give conflicting stories or can give no reason for the injury ("he woke up from his nap and couldn't move his arms. I don't know what happened"). Parents who are unaware that certain conduct is extreme behavior—such as holding a child's hand over an open flame to teach him not to touch the stove again—will describe their action as part of giving a routine history.

Listen for points in the history that are not only inconsistent between caregivers, but inconsistent with the injury, such as the child has fresh ecchymotic marks (bright red), but the parent says they are from a fall a week ago, or the parent reports that all that happened was that the child rolled off the couch, but now the child has two broken arms. Listen for accounts of abnormal development in the history that don't seem plausible, such as a parent reporting that a 6-month-old child crawled up onto a stove and burned himself. Blaming an injury on a younger sibling is also common. Evaluate whether such a happening sounds as if it could have actually happened.

To prevent continuing abuse from such parents, children may assume a role reversal with their parents or become the comforting, solacing person. When questioned about the injury, abused children often repeat the parent's story; this loyalty to parents seems misplaced, but they may fear further beatings if they say otherwise. Do not assume, therefore, that because the child says no abuse has occurred that this is necessarily true.

Allowing young children to play with anatomically correct dolls is a method of allowing children who have been sexually abused to describe what happened to them. Recounting sexual abuse is very difficult for young children. They may have been told not to tell anyone about the abuse, or they may not have the vocabulary to be able to name body parts to express themselves clearly.

Physical Examination

Children should be completely undressed for a physical exam so that every part of their body can be inspected. Bandaids should be removed and the skin underneath inspected. Ecchymotic marks typically appear red to purple immediately after an injury, then progress through green (the 5th to 7th day), yellow (the 7th to 10th day), and brown (the 10th to 14th days). They clear by about 15 days following the injury. Describing the color of these marks, therefore, dates the injury. Height and weight are important assessments to plot, as these measurements may be delayed in abused and neglected children.

A number of injuries clearly signal abuse. Adult human bites or missing chunks of hair rarely occur by accident (Kornberg, 1992). Children who are beaten with electrical cords, belts, or clotheslines have peculiar circular or looped lesions. Children beaten with a belt buckle have additional curved lacerations from the imprint of the buckle. Abrasions or ecchymotic areas on the wrists or ankles may be present if a child was tied to a bed or a wall. Ecchymotic lesions at the sides of the mouth may mark where a gag was applied. Most parents protect their children's hands carefully from injury. An injury to the hands is therefore suspect of abuse (Johnson, Kaufman, & Callendar, 1990). Bruised areas on the ulnar surface of the forearm suggest that a child used a defensive posture to ward off an attack. Retinal hemorrhages may indicate abusive shaking, particularly in infants.

Burns or scalds occur in about 10% of abused children. When children burn their hands by accident, they usually burn the palm; burns from abuse are often on the dorsal surface. Young children do accidentally step into bathtubs containing water that is hot enough to burn. When this happens, however, the child usually falls forward and so also has burns on the hands and splash marks on the chest or face. When a child is lowered into scalding water as punishment, only the feet and skin up to the knees are scalded, with a sharp demarcation of normal tissue. A child placed in a tub of hot water, buttocks first, often has no burn in the center of his buttocks because the buttocks touched the tub; a ring of burns causing a "hole in the doughnut" effect appears around this (Hobbs, 1989).

Cigarette burns are a common finding on the bodies of physically abused children. A fresh cigarette burn causes a blister that resembles the scab of impetigo (Rogosta, 1989). Differentiation at this stage is often difficult. Impetigo lesions, however, heal without scarring. Cigarette burns heal with a definite circular scar.

A sexually transmitted disease in a young girl or an isolated post-fourchette injury in a preadolescent suggests sexual abuse (DeJong, 1992). X-ray findings of fractures at different ages of healing, rib and long bone fractures in infants, scapulae and sternal fractures without a specific history, and skull fractures more severe than linear in infants are diagnostic (Wissow, 1990).

A number of child care practices can simulate abuse. Cupping is a Russian and Eastern European therapy used to treat pain. In this practice, a cup or glass is heated and placed over a skin area to relieve pain. This results in round, well marked erythematous areas (Asner & Wisotsky, 1981). Coin rolling (*cao gio*) is a far eastern practice used to treat fever, headache, or chills. Oil is applied to the chest or back and then a coin is rubbed against the skin. Sharply bordered, bilateral symmetric petechiae or purpura lines are left on the skin (Rosenblat & Hong, 1989). Both these practices, although probably not effective, are harmless and should not be mistaken for child abuse.

Discharge Instructions

When reviewing discharge instructions with parents, parental neglect may be first suspected. A parent who states that he or she does not intend to fill an antibiotic prescription because the injury was the child's fault and he deserves an infection, or a parent who states that he or she has no intention of returning for follow-up care, might be examples of this.

ISSUES OF CHILD ABUSE REPORTING

As nurses become more involved in child abuse reporting, a number of important controversies arise.

Isn't Reporting Child Abuse Unethical as it Violates Nurse/Client Confidentiality?

It is true that the second standard of the American Nurses Association (ANA) Code of Ethics states "the nurse safeguards the client's right to privacy by judiciously protecting information of a confidential nature" (American Nurses Association [ANA], 1985).

Based on this, a report of child abuse does break the elementary contract for confidentiality between clients and nurses. The law is aware of this contradiction, however, and following a philosophy of preventing a greater evil, allows the contradiction to exist in the interest of children's welfare.

Are Only Pediatric Nurses Involved in the Problem?

The usual health care setting where child abuse is revealed is an emergency room. This means that emergency room personnel (not necessarily child health nurses) are prime people to recognize and report child abuse. Adult practitioners in other areas are not immune, as abuse is sometimes discovered by a parent's statement to a psychiatric clinician or adult care nurse, such as "I shook him to make him stop crying" or "I have to get home. The children aren't safe with my boyfriend." In many instances in which a woman in the family is being battered, a child is being abused as well (McKibben, De Vos, & Newberger, 1989). An adult practitioner caring for abused women, therefore, might become aware of the problem, and if child abuse is suspected, must file a report. A pedophile (an adult who seeks out children for sexual gratification) might admit during therapy that he is still abusing children. This poses a severe ethical quandary for nurses, and knowing that child abuse will be reported this way can prevent pedophiles from coming for counseling.

A maternal-newborn nurse might become aware that abuse seems likely during the postpartal period when he or she observes a mother demonstrating no interest in a newborn or treating her newborn in an emotionally abusive manner.

School nurses can become aware of a child who is dressed improperly for the weather (neglect) or has physical marks of abuse. As teachers in most states are also designated as mandated reporters of abuse, school administrators have a system in place similar to that in hospitals, where one central school official is designated as the person to file the abuse report.

Will Reporting Abuse Further Endanger the Child
by Making the Parents Angry at the Child?

Some fear that reporting abuse will actually bring increased trauma to a child by initiating increased abuse by a parent, because he or she is angry that the child has admitted to abuse. There is also a concern that the report will subject the child to increased stress by having the family stigmatized as an abusing one and the child forced to testify against a parent in court.

Courts are becoming aware that asking a child to testify against a parent is a stressful situation. Ways that courts have tried to reduce this trauma are: exclusion of spectators from the courtroom; videotaping of the child's testimony to avoid direct confrontation between the child and the abuser; taping the child's statement to avoid the child having to repeat the story to differing attorneys or child care agency personnel, provision of a court appointed advocate for the child, and the allowance of hearsay testimony (a physician repeating the child's story rather than the child having to do this) (Whitcomb, Shapiro, & Stellwagen, 1985). Not all states have these provisions in place, because the right to face an accuser directly in court is a constitutional right; hearsay evidence is generally not admissible.

Reporting Abuse is Dangerous as it Can Bring Legal Retaliation Against the Nurse

As discussed, abuse reporting laws are written with an *immunity* provision, this guarantees that the reporter can not be prosecuted for the report if the report later proves to be false, as long as the report was made in "good faith." It is important for nurses to record their observations in the child's chart in a way that assures there can be no doubt of "good faith." A statement such as "parents were rude to emergency room personnel while ecchymotic areas on child were being examined" is inappropriate, as it suggests a nurse was more interested in revenge than objective reporting.

Isn't it Dangerous to Confront Suspected Abusive Parents with Suspicion of Abuse, as They may Retaliate with Abusive Behavior Against the Nurse?

Following the official report of suspected abuse, it is the responsibility of a member of the health care team to inform the parents that a suspicion of child abuse has been raised and the official report has been filed. This is part of establishing a truthful relationship with the parents. This role could fall to a nurse practitioner or clinician. It is important in these instances for a nurse to limit the exchange to factual information. State the reason for the report ("your child has injuries that can not be explained by your history") followed by an explanation of what will happen next ("the child will be admitted to the hospital; a social worker will call on you in one or two days"). This is not the time to try and force parents to admit guilt (they may not be guilty or the parent who brought in the child may not be the guilty one) or to try and make them say they are sorry the abuse occurred. Trying to provoke this type of response can lead to controversy about the report and perhaps abusive behavior toward the nurse.

Are Nurses Responsible Child Abuse Reporters?

Nurses have a minimal track record in actually filing abuse reports, as in many instances in the past this responsibility has been passed to a hospital official. There is no reason, however, to suspect that nurses who assume responsible practice positions will do this less well than other mandated reporters. In a national survey conducted to estimate the rate of noncompliant reporting, Zellman (1991) found that as many as 40% of mandated reporters stated they were guilty of having been in noncompliance of reporting or had not reported suspected abuse at some time.

New York State mandated in 1990 that all registered nurses, along with other mandated abuse reporters, complete a 2-hour course on child abuse before they would be eligible to renew their professional licenses. A total of 253 nurses who enrolled at classes taught at the State University of New York at Buffalo were asked to complete a questionnaire regarding abuse reporting to determine their ability to objectively report abuse. Ninety percent of this study sample was female, with ages ranging from 24 to 52 years. Only 10% of these nurses indicated that they had ever made a report of child maltreatment or neglect over the last 2 years.

The questionnaire for the study contained two short vignettes depicting children with common symptoms of possible child abuse and one vignette depicting a child with symptoms more reflective of leukemia than abuse. During administration, the vignettes were held constant as to the abuse situation, while the socioeconomic level of the family was systematically varied so that at different times, the families represented upper-, middle-, or lower-class backgrounds. Participants in the study were asked to read each vignette and then indicate on a five-point Lickert scale if, based on the information provided, they would suspect abuse enough to report it.

Findings from the study revealed that 84.8% of the participating nurses indicated that they would report abuse when the family was depicted as being from a high socioeconomic background; 80% stated that they would report abuse when the family was depicted as being from a low socioeconomic background. There is no significant difference between these two findings. In contrast, when the family was depicted as being from a middle income background or that most like the nurses themselves, only 54.6% of participants indicated that they would report abuse (a significant difference from the first two findings, $p = <.01$). In this same study, 87% of nurses indicated that they would report abuse when the victim was male; only 54.7% indicated that they would report abuse when the victim was a female. This is, again, a significant difference ($p = >.01$) (Pillitteri, Seidl, Smith, & Stanton, 1992). Zellman (1991) suggests that such a difference in reporting abuse more for male than female infants occurs because male infants are more valued than female infants by Western society.

The implication of this study is that if nurses carry this projected reporting ability into actual practice, nurses may fail to report child abuse when the victim is female or from a middle-class family, but report it when the victim is from another socioeconomic level.

Did respondents in the study cited above overreport child abuse? The symptoms of the child in the third vignette included symptoms more representative of a blood dyscrasia (swollen glands, rhinitis, bleeding gums) than child abuse. Sixty-nine percent of participants stated they would report abuse based on this vignette. This finding is equal to the number of respondents who reported that they would report the two vignettes designed to represent child abuse (69.4% compared to 70.1%) (Pillitteri, et al, 1992).

As nurses become more active reporters, they are well advised to monitor their responses to suspicions of child abuse so they can be certain they are objective child abuse reporters and not overly influenced by the child's gender or the family's socioeconomic standing and that they make appropriate referrals for further diagnostic workups if they are called for.

What if the Abuse Occurred in the Past and is no Longer Occurring?

Most states do not have a statute of limitations for child abuse, or there is no time frame after which the offender is free from blame. Reporting this type of abuse calls for judgement based on whether there is a possibility the offender still has contact with the child and or other children or if the child is an adolescent.

Does Charting Suspected Child Abuse Call for Special Techniques?

Charting to document suspected child abuse requires the same careful charting techniques necessary for any health care contact.

Quote the child's statement about his or her injuries exactly and put quotation marks around the words to show they are a direct quote. Make it clear whether the child's statement was something said spontaneously or in answer to a question (cite the question that initiated the statement if this is so).

Be certain that notes contain statements, not conclusions ("mother's breath smelled of alcohol and she walked unsteadily," *not*, "she was in-

toxicated"). Because a chart can be used in court as evidence it is important that observations be recorded accurately but, also so they can be
interpreted by a nonmedical person, such as a judge. To be certain the
note is clear, limit the use of abbreviations so that nonmedical personnel can easily understand them (not "WNWPWM" but "well-nourished,
well-proportioned white male"). Describing an area as "ecchymotic" may
not be as helpful as calling a mark a "bruise" (or follow "ecchymotic area"
by "bruise"). If an injury is in the shape of a specific object (if J-shaped
marks of a belt buckle are present, for example) or the imprint of teeth is
present, don't be reluctant to state that the appearance is that of a buckle
or teeth marks.

The taking of photographs is indispensable in documenting the existence and appearance of bruises or burns. If assisting with these, be certain the room is well lighted; ask the photographer to include a color
marker at the size of the photograph, so that the color of bruises can be
duplicated on developing, and lay a ruler next to a lesion to validate its
size. Photographs should include two views: one close up and one at a
distance to document the position of the lesion on the child's body
(Smistek, 1992).

If Polaroid photographs are added to a record, be certain they are taped
to a chart page, not merely paper-clipped in place, as the chart will pass
through many hands over the next few months.

Isn't Using Nurses' Time for Child Abuse Reporting an Unwise Use of Nursing Time?

Filling in forms is rarely viewed as an effective use of nurses' time. As
nursing practice increases in autonomy and scope, however, administrative responsibilities that must be assumed also increase. In those instances when a nurse is the sole health care provider for a child and therefore the sole person able to suspect abuse, taking the time to fill out the
report is an important part of providing care and safeguarding the child's
health. Being named as mandated reporters of child abuse is not meant
to increase nurses' paperwork time, but shows society's recognition of
nurses' competence and ability to carry out this function. Finally, it re-
spects the important role of nurses as client advocates.

TOPICS FOR DISCUSSION

1. Suppose you assessed the child of a prominent person in your community (Such as the mayor or a clergyman) and suspected that the
   marks present on the child suggest child abuse? Would knowing the

parents are well-known and respected in the community make abuse more difficult to report?

2. Suppose you are working as a school nurse and a child tells you he has not been fed for 3 days. A brother says that isn't true. What would you do? Trust the brother? Report this child as neglected?

3. Suppose a 14-year-old boy tells you he is being sexually molested by a stepfather but then begs you not to tell anyone? What would you do? Would your action be different if the child were a girl?

4. Suppose a 16-year-old client you are caring for tells you that he was sexually abused by her father from the time she was 7 until she was 12 (when her parents were divorced and he left the home). Would you report this? Does it make a difference that the abuse is no longer occurring?

REFERENCES

American Nurses Association. (1985). *Code for Nurses*. Kansas City, MO: Author.

Asner, R. S., & Wisotsky, D. H. (1981). Cupping lesions simulating child abuse. *Journal of Pediatrics, 99*, 267–268.

Caffey, J. (1946). Multiple fractures in the long bones of infants suffering from chronic subdural hematoma. *American Journal of Radiology, 56*, 163–166.

DeJong, A. R. (1992). Genital and anal trauma. In S. Ludwig, and A. E. Kornberg (Eds.) *Child abuse* (2nd ed., pp. 131–247). NY: Churchill Livingstone.

Dobbs, D. (1986). Legal responsibilities and liabilities when treating child abuse. *Pediatric Emergency Care, 2*, 40–43.

Gil, D. (1971). Violence against children. *Journal of Marriage and the Family, 33*, 637–640.

Hobbs, C. J. (1989). ABC of child abuse: Burns and scalds. *British Medical Journal, 298*, 1302–1305.

Johnson, C. F., Kaufman, K. L., & Callendar, C. (1990). The hand as a target organ in child abuse. *Clinical Pediatrics, 29*, 66–72.

Kempe, C. H., Silverman, F. N., Steele, B. F., Droegmueller, W., & Silver, H. K. (1962). The battered child syndrome. *Journal of the American Medical Association, 181*, 17–24.

Kornberg, A. E. (1992). Recognizing and reporting child abuse. In S. Ludwig and A. E. Kornberg (Eds.) *Child abuse* (2nd ed., pp. 13–24). NY: Churchill Livingstone.

Lazoritz, S. (1990). Whatever happened to Mary Ellen? *Child Abuse and Neglect, 14*, 143–145.

Lazoritz, S. (1992). Child abuse: An historical perspective. In S. Ludwig & A. E. Kornberg (Eds.), *Child abuse* (2nd ed., pp. 85–90). New York: Churchill Livingstone.

McKibben, L., De Vos, E., & Newberger, E. H. (1989). Victimization of mothers of abused children: A controlled study. *Pediatrics, 84*, 531–535.

Pillitteri, A. (1993). Paper presented at conference, Child Abuse, Historical Analysis of Child Abuse and Neglect. Buffalo, NY. State University of New York at Buffalo.

Pillitteri, A., Seidl, A., Smith, C., & Stanton, M. (1992). Parent gender, victim gender and family socioeconomic level influences on the potential reporting of physical abuse by nurses. *Issues in Comprehensive Pediatric Nursing, 16*, 387–392.

Rogosta, K. (1989). Pediculosis masquerades as child abuse. *Pediatric Emergency Care, 5*, 253–354.

Rosenblat, J., & Hong, P. (1989). Coin rolling misdiagnosed as child abuse. *Canadian Medical Association Journal, 140*, 417–420.

Schetky, D. H. (1986). Emerging issues in child sexual abuse. *Journal of the American Academy of Child Psychology, 25*, 490–492.

Senner, A., & Ott, M. J. (1989). Munchausen syndrome by proxy. *Issues in Comprehensive Pediatric Nursing, 12*, 345–357.

Smistek, B. S. (1992). Photography of the abused and neglected child. In S. Ludwig & A. E. Kornberg (Eds.), *Child abuse* (2nd ed., pp. 467–477). New York: Churchill Livingstone.

Spaide, R. F., Swengel, R. M., & Mein, C. E. (1990). Shaken baby syndrome. *American Family Physician, 41*, 1145–1151.

Straus, M. A., & Gelles, R. J. (1990). *Behind closed doors: Violence in the American family.* Garden City: Anchor Press.

Whitcomb, D., Shapiro, E. R., & Stellwagen, L. D. (1985). *When the victim is a child: Issues for judges and prosecutors.* Washington, D.C.: U.S. Government Printing Office.

Wissow, L. S. (1990). Epidemiology and definitions. In L. S. Wissow (Ed.), *Child advocacy for the clinician* (pp. 1–11). Baltimore: Williams & Wilkins.

Wong, D. L. (1987). False allegations of child abuse: The other side of the tragedy. *Pediatric Nursing, 13*, 329–333.

Zellman, G. L. (1991). Report decision-making patterns among mandated child abuse reporters. *Child Abuse & Neglect, 14*, 325–336.

8

Adolescent Pregnancy and Sexual Activity

Mattie L. Rhodes

Though recent years have shown some decline and stabilization in the pregnancy rate, adolescent pregnancy and sexual activity remain at epidemic proportions. More than one million teenage girls in the United States become pregnant each year. One out of every 10 girls aged 15–19 becomes pregnant (Henshaw and Van Vort, 1989; Pratt, Mosher, Bachrach, & Harn, 1984). In 1985, 31,000 of the 1.03 million pregnant teenagers were younger than 15; and 850,000 were aged 15–19. In 1990, there were 23,000 pregnancies among women 14 and younger (Hatcher et al., 1990). Pregnancy outcomes for the one million teenage girls included 477,710 live births and 416,710 induced abortions, the rest were miscarriages and still births (Trussell, 1988).

Girls under age 15 in the United States are at least five times as likely to give birth as young adolescents in any developed country, even though initiation of sex among this population is similar. Part of this difference may be related to the reluctance of American society to support the use of contraceptives by teenagers. Data from the third cycle of the National Survey of Family Growth in 1982 indicated that approximately 30% of never-married 15–19-year-old women were not practicing contraception (Bachrach, 1984).

The total number of pregnancies change as the adolescent population changes. The population of youths aged 15 to 24 is expected to decline from 43 million to 34 million by 1996 (Wetzel, 1987). Adolescent pregnancies reached a high point in 1980 and thereafter experienced some fluctuations with a slight downward trend (Forrest & Singh, 1990) (see Table 8.1).

The trend in overall birth rates for ages 15–19 reveal the same fluctuation patterns as the pregnancy rates (see Table 8.2).

110

TABLE 8.1 Pregnancy Rate per 1000 Females Aged 15–19

1977	1979	1981	1983	1985
104.6	109.4	110.8	109.9	109.8

From "Advanced Report on Final Natality Statistics 1985," *Monthly Vital Statistics Report, 36*, Supplement, 1987.

Births for ages 18–19 were the highest, showing a decline until 1986 when there was a slight rise. For the very young, aged 10–14, births declined after 1970 and increased after 1986. There is much concern for any pregnancy and birth for this very young population, since problems are particularly acute for them.

SEXUAL ACTIVITY

Many researchers have reported a trend of increased permissiveness toward premarital sexual activity. This applies to both males and females. There appeared to be a sexual revolution in the late 1960s and early 1970s, leveling off in the late seventies. This increase was first noted among the older teenagers aged 18–19 and spread to those younger (Hofferth, Kahn & Baldwin, 1987). These younger teenagers aged 10–14 are engaging in

TABLE 8.2 Birthrate by Age and Race Per 1000 Females Aged 10–19, 1960–1986

Age	1960	1970	1980	1983	1986
15–19					
Total	89.1	68.3	53.0	51.7	50.6
White	79.4	57.4	44.7	43.6	41.8
Black	156.1	147.7	100.0	95.5	98.1
18–19					
Total	—	114.7	82.1	78.1	81.0
White	—	101.5	72.1	68.3	69.8
Black	—	204.9	138.8	130.4	141.0
15–17					
Total	—	38.8	32.5	32.0	30.6
White	—	29.2	25.2	24.8	23.4
Black	—	101.4	73.6	70.1	70.0
10–14					
Total	0.8	1.2	1.1	1.1	1.3
White	0.4	0.5	0.6	0.6	0.6
Black	4.3	5.2	4.3	4.1	4.6

From National Center for Health Statistics Advance Report of Final Natality Statistics, 1986; *Monthly Vital Statistics Report.* Vol. 37, No 3 Supplement 1988, Table 18, p. 32. U.S. Bureau of Census, *Statistical Abstracts of the United States*, 1992.

sexual activity in increasing proportions, and generally the consequences are more serious. Some 4.2 million women aged 15–19 have had intercourse at least once (Trussell, 1988). About half of women aged 15–19 in metropolitan areas are sexually active (Mosher, 1990). The trend shows that sexual activity (intercourse) for ages 15–19 increased from 28.6% in 1970 to 51.5% in 1988. During the years from 1970–1988, adolescent women who reported having premarital sexual activity increased by at least 55% (National Center for Health Statistics (NCHS), 1990). The largest increase, however, occurred among those aged 15 years.

SOCIAL ANTECEDENTS OF PREGNANCY AND SEXUAL ACTIVITY

Adolescent pregnancy and parenthood is not just a minority problem or one only of poor youth. In 1985 there were 323,000 births to white adolescents 140,000 to Black adolescents, and 62,000 to Hispanic adolescents. However, a large proportion of the teens who become pregnant are poor and from disadvantaged backgrounds (Chilman, 1980; Pittman & Adams, 1988; Trussell, 1988). There are increased proportions of Blacks and Hispanics who are from lower socioeconomic status. This lower SES is associated with disadvantaged educational and economic backgrounds, fewer opportunities to fulfill career aspirations, and dismal life options. Findings from a national longitudinal survey of youth conducted in 1982 indicate that Blacks and hispanics generally have less favorable educational backgrounds and lower labor force participation. Compared to white adolescents, Blacks are four times as likely and Hispanics are two times as likely to have given birth by age 18. Rates of sexual activity are higher for Blacks than whites, while Hispanics are somewhere in the middle of the two (Children's Defense Fund, 1988).

Adolescents raised in impoverished environments are at greater risk for participating in pregnancy-risking behaviors than those raised in more affluent environments. The culture of poverty (Lewis, 1966) produces social structural conditions which give rise to disorganization of individual attitudes, beliefs and values, bringing about feelings of despair, helplessness, low self-esteem, and an inability to defer sexual gratification. This impoverishment is transmitted from generation to generation, rendering children helpless to adequately take advantage of opportunities in their lives. Poverty has also been related to feelings of low self-esteem, hopelessness, and fatalism in reference to future educational or occupational aspirations (Stack, 1974; Staples, 1973). These feelings are highly correlated with early sexual activity and pregnancy.

Teenagers overall are less likely to use contraceptives than are older persons. Black adolescents are less likely to use contraceptives than Hispanics, with white adolescents the most likely to practice contraceptive behavior. This increased tendency to use contraceptives accounts somewhat for lower pregnancy rates among whites (Bachrach, 1984).

Poverty is a major factor in this myriad of problems. Some researchers have found that Blacks living in middle-class neighborhoods with better school systems and more resources have lower rates of sexual activity, pregnancy, and births than their counterparts in lower socioeconomic environments (Furstenberg, 1987; Hogan & Kitagawa, 1985). American Indians, Hispanics, and Blacks from higher socioeconomic environments have fewer births than their lower SES counterparts (Franklin, 1988).

FAMILY INFLUENCES

The family, the primary social unit, is important as a socialization structure for the individual. The behavior of the adolescent is the product of the social elements in the environment, with the family an important part of that environment. Many family members—mother, father, and siblings—play a significant role in the development of the adolescent's behavior. The mother generally has the major responsibility for domestic and socioemotional functions in managing the house, as well as increased interaction with the children. The mother's influence over the child's life tends to dominate that of the father. In situations where the father is absent a large part of the day working, and the mother works at home, the father has a limited, indirect kind of power, since the family is dependent on his economic pursuits. In general, however, the father is still more available to the mother for emotional support, as well as some participation in family decisionmaking and sharing of some of the family responsibilities, than in female-headed households. Interactions between father and mother are important in making day-to-day decisions regarding the family. Adolescents in these situations have the advantage of both their mother's and father's emotional support. In nuclear, intact families when the wife is employed outside the home, the mother's contact with children may begin to approximate that of the father's. The husband and wife in these situations may have more egalitarian roles related to managing the household and raising the children.

Single-parent households are different from these traditional families. Adolescents in these settings have different experiences. The most common single-parent arrangement is the female-headed. Adolescents in single-parent female-headed households are at high risk for pregnancy-risking behavior, including early dating and early sexual activity. From 1970 to 1983 the number of one-parent families with children increased 107% (U.S. Department of Commerce, 1983). Currently, one out of five, or approximately 11 million children, live in single-parent homes (Children's Defense Fund, 1985). Income in female-headed households is likely to be low.

Single-parent units differ from the traditional family unit in other ways, including general function, types of stress, ways of coping with stress, income resources, and support systems. Such mothers suffer from work overload in trying to perform the functions of both parents in meeting the needs of the family. Women in these types of situations are more likely to have problems related to economic and household management (Epstein, 1979). These parents have fewer resources to provide educational and career opportunities for their children.

In 1984 families maintained by women accounted for 16% of all families and 48% of poor families (U.S. Census Bureau, 1985). In 1986 46% of Black children were living in households with incomes below the poverty line, as compared to 17.7% of white children. In 1987, the mean family income of female-headed households was $15,419, in contrast to $37,092 for married-couple families (U.S. Census Bureau, 1990). These types of salaries do not allow for the child care needed between the times that the child gets home from school and the mother gets home from work. Thus adult absence may be a problem, with the child left alone to make decisions that are beyond the scope of his or her experience. In these female-headed households, the mother serves as a role model for female children. These teens may receive the message that single-parent household arrangements are the norm. Mothers of pregnant teenagers were often teenage mothers themselves (Furstenberg & Crawford, 1978). This is not favorable modeling behavior desired for these teenagers.

CONSEQUENCES OF ADOLESCENT PREGNANCY

Early pregnancy in teenagers often has unfortunate social and psychological consequences. Early parenthood and childbearing diminishes the ability of the young adolescent to achieve educational goals. The added responsibilities related to child care takes away time and effort needed to focus on educational pursuits. These mothers are much more likely to drop out of high school even when compared to peers of similar socioeconomic backgrounds and academic aptitude (Card & Wise, 1981). This remains true even though some cities allow pregnant adolescents to continue to attend regular school if they desire. This disruption is sometimes permanent.

Teenage mothers and fathers are less likely to find stable employment, partially due to their lack of skills and disadvantaged academic backgrounds, and therefore are more likely to rely on public assistance than men and women who begin childbearing later in life (Hofferth & Moore, 1979). Some argue that adolescent mothers had low academic histories and goals before pregnancy occurred, which may have been part of the reason they risked pregnancy in the first place. Pregnancy may have also been the primary cause of dropping out of school.

Early sexual involvement increases the risk not only of early pregnancy but of sexually transmitted diseases as well. Sexually transmitted diseases (STDs) are infectious diseases transmitted through sexual contact. They include more than 20 different organisms and diagnoses. Adolescents, compared with older age groups, have higher rates of gonorrhea and chlamydia, and these diseases, if untreated, can lead to pelvic inflammatory disease (PID). The consequences of PID can include infertility and ectopic pregnancy. HIV virus (human immunodeficiency virus) causes a defect in the body's immune system by invading and then multiplying in the body's white cells. AIDS occurs when the HIV-infected person develops symptoms. As of now, this disease is fatal. The risk of transmission is high through sexual contact with an infected partner. The AIDS virus has been identified in blood, semen, and vaginal secretions, and can be transmitted from the body of an infected person through a portal of entry into another person, usually a sexual partner.

Genital warts, caused by the human papilloma virus (HPV) is one of the most common viral STDs in the U.S. (Hatcher et al, 1990). Spread of this virus is directly related to early onset of sexual activity and multiple sexual partners. These warts appear as single or multiple soft fleshy growths around the anus, vulvovaginal area, penis, urethra, or perineum. Certain strains of the HPV have been associated with cervical cancer.

Herpes virus types 1 and 2 are of serious concern also. There is no cure for this infection, manifested by vesicular lesions in the genitalia leading to contagious painful lesions in areas of contact, that is, the genitals and oral cavities.

Teenage mothers are at high risk of premature or stillborn birth and of birth defects resulting from poor prenatal care and poor follow-up compliance. The impact of the birth event on the body of a teenage female is a tremendous physical occurrence. There is concern whether the teenage body has reached the physical maturity needed for a successful reproductive process. At all stages of pregnancy and infancy, the very young mother is a greater risk for infant mortality and prematurity. Unmarried Blacks and the disadvantaged run the greatest risk of these problems, since they are more likely to be of lower socioeconomic status and receive little or no prenatal care. Premature infants are at greatest risk for health conditions as epilepsy, cerebral palsy and mental retardation, deafness, blindness, and other physical problems related to immature physical and mental development.

SOLUTIONS TO THE PROBLEM

Delay Sexual Gratification

Encourage adolescents to avoid sexual activity by delaying sexual gratification. Educate teens regarding the alternatives involved in making sexual decisions. These programs should emphasize responsible sexual behavior. Many such programs exist today. Teenagers with high educational aspirations, high academic performance, and future aspirations are more likely to avoid sexual involvement if they feel there is a chance of it interfering in their future career plans. Focus on information that provides an understanding regarding factors leading to premature sexual activity. This education should focus on the many risks of early sexual involvement: health risks, guilt feelings, lower self-esteem, and feelings of being used. Encourage teens to practice abstinence by saying no. Not only should programs encourage abstinence, but they should also offer alternatives to sexual involvement for teens. The American Family Life Act passed by Congress in 1981 stressed teaching teens to abstain until marriage. This same act provided about $10–$15 million per year to programs promoting self-control and alternatives.

Encourage Use of Contraceptives Among Adolescents who are Sexually Active or at High-risk

With the increase in sexual behavior among teenagers, it is unrealistic to expect that stressing abstinence will be successful in all cases. The legitimation of contraceptive use among sexually active teenagers is a reasonable approach. If close to half of the nation's teenagers are sexually active, then it seems reasonable to provide information and contraceptive services, and to educate teenagers regarding their effective use. Less than half of sexually active teenagers used any form of birth control. The preferred methods used by this group are the pill and condom (Rhodes, 1992). This brings up the issue of parental involvement in decisions related to the procurement and use of contraceptives and contraceptive education and counseling. A growing number of advocates support availability of contraceptive services without parental consent. In most states, over-the-counter contraceptives are available to teenagers without parental consent, and in some states, New York included, clinics treat teenagers without parental consent.

Within this arena, education should be provided regarding the responsibilities related to contraceptive use. In many cases, this would require a change in thinking in American society. Other countries make both contraceptives and counseling services more available to this age group. Some feel that schools should be involved in this effort, while others argue that a school-linked approach is not the answer. One such program was evaluated in several schools in Baltimore (Zabin, Hirsch, Smith, Emerson, King, Street, & Hardy, 1988). In this program, sex education and counseling services were offered in pilot schools. After 28 months of operation, results showed a decrease in pregnancy rate in these schools. Though this seems to lend support to the concept of a school-based contraceptive program, these results were based only on a small sample of the population, and therefore may have limited application to the general population.

In order to protect against sexually transmitted diseases, teens need to have barrier protection. Barrier protection involves use of some kind of mechanical device to prevent passage of sperm into the body of the sexual partner.

Mechanical barriers available to women include diaphragms, cervical caps, and sponges. Diaphragms and cervical caps require the use of contraceptive jelly (spermicides). Advantages include: (1) high effectiveness from pregnancy; (2) significant protection against sexually transmitted diseases; (3) medical safety; and (4) very low failure rates. Disadvantages of these include: (1) they are available only by prescription; (2) they need to be fitted by a health care provider, and (3) they require advanced planning, since insertion is necessary before intercourse. The sponge, sold over the counter, is not as effective.

The condom is a male barrier contraceptive. The condom provides better protection from both pregnancy and STDs than do other contraceptives. The use of both the condom and a spermicide offers the most protection from both pregnancy and STDs. Spermicides immobilize sperm; most have an active ingredient, nonoxynol-9, which serves also to kill the sperm. Nonoxynol-9 has also been shown to offer significant protection against organisms causing gonorrhea, chlamydia, genital herpes, trichomonas, and, in some cases, AIDS (Can you rely on Condoms?, 1989). Generally, if used properly, spermicides are quite effective. It is reasonable to combine the use of the condom with any other types of contraceptive such as birth control pills. Oral contraceptives protect only against pregnancy, not AIDS or other STDs. When condoms or diaphragms are used a spermicide containing nonxynol-9 is necessary, since diaphragms alone do not provide enough protection from transmission of the AIDS virus. The combination of spermicides (a chemical barrier) and a condom (a mechanical barrier) offer the most effective protection against transmission of the AIDS virus and most of the STDs.

It is important for teens to be properly educated and skilled regarding the use of condoms, and it is realistic to plan to teach and demonstrate to teens how to properly apply condoms. Contraceptive counseling and services should be made available by trained professionals at low or no cost to teenagers desiring them, especially those high-risk sexually active teens. Contraceptives for teens should be accessible, affordable, safe, and effective for the purposes intended as well as easy to use. Methods which require a prescription from the physician can be an obstacle that teens are not willing to overcome. Much controversy centers around the ethics of contraception for minors (teenagers). Should teens be allowed the freedom to control matters related to their own bodies and parenthood, or should it be done with knowledge and consent of parents?

Enhance the Options Available to High-risk Disadvantaged Adolescents

This includes early intervention in the lives of socioeconomically deprived adolescents. Enhanced socioeconomic conditions and better educational resources early on in life to provide a solid foundation in basic skills from which to build.

More positive role models should be made available for children from disadvantaged ghetto environments. In most cases, these adolescents are exposed to adults whom they respect and love who have similar backgrounds and similar behavior all resulting from residing in impoverished neighborhoods. These teenagers should be exposed to positive progressive role models who are genuinely interested in their well-being and welfare.

Improve employment programs for disadvantaged populations. These programs should not only provide jobs, but should also prepare the teenager with job readiness skills.

ROLE OF THE NURSE

Nurses have a key role in the prevention of unwanted teenage pregnancies and STDs. Nurses working in the community should encourage primary prevention by working with parents and adolescents. The nurse should be prepared to make careful assessments of adolescents who are at risk for sexual activity and/or pregnancy. Support for community leaders and parents should be encouraged. These groups should be educated regarding issues related to this population. Educational programs should focus on 1) normal adolescent sexual development; 2) sexually transmitted diseases; and 3) pregnancy-preventive behavior, including abstinence as well as contraceptive techniques. These programs can be presented to adolescents as well as parents.

Input from the adolescent, the parent, and community leaders regarding program strategies should be sought. Parents, school officials, and community leaders should be informed about community-based clinics for adolescents. These clinics are in place around the country, with positive results. Community and school nurses can encourage school officials to include sex education in their curricula early in the school experience. Nurses can make very significant contributions to program design and content and also assist in the education of teachers.

Nurses in the clinic setting should be prepared to provide counseling for adolescents. It is important that this counseling be done in a setting that is confidential and attractive to this population. The nurse should establish rapport with the adolescents so that open discussions can occur. This is also an opportunity for the nurse to answer questions and provide clarification. The location of the clinic should be such that the adolescent feels comfortable attending. Preferably the clinic should provide a variety of services to give a sense of confidentiality as to services are being sought. Nurses working in these settings should be prepared to be advocates for adolescents in need.

Nurse practitioners, clinicians, and university nurse faculty members should be involved in conducting intervention and evaluation research on issues related to adolescents, and be willing to share this information with colleagues. This research can be used to design staff development programs based on adolescent needs. Nurse educators have a responsibility to prepare students adequately to deal with adolescent sexuality issues.

TOPICS FOR DISCUSSION

1. How do you explain the fact that the teenage pregnancy rate is higher in the United States than in the other developed countries?
2. At what age should sex education in the schools start? What should the content be in the early classes?
3. In what ways can nurses participate in the sex education program in schools?
4. Given the current epidemic of sexually transmitted diseases, what type of contraceptives do you suggest for teenagers?

5. What are the advantages and disadvantages of establishing separate clinics for teenagers?
6. If you were called upon to teach a series of guest lectures on sexuality to teenagers, what content would you include?
7. If one of the parents called you up the day before your first guest lecture and told you that you should make your primary focus abstinence education (and say nothing about contraception) how would you handle the situation?

REFERENCES

Bachrach, C. A. (1984). Contraceptive practice among American women, 1973–1982. *Family Planning Perspective, 16*, 253–259.

Bullough, V., & Bullough, B. (1990). *Contraception: A guide to birth control methods*. Buffalo, New York: Prometheus Books.

Can you rely on condoms? (1989, March). *Consumer Reports, 54*, 136, 141.

Card, J. J., & Wise, L. L. (1978). Teenage mothers and teenage fathers: The impact of early childbearing on the parents' personal and professional lives. *Family Planning Perspectives, 10*, 199–205.

Children's Defense Fund. (1988). *Teenage pregnancy: An advocate's guide to the numbers*. Publication of the Adolescent Prevention Clearinghouse, CDF, 122 C St., NW, Washington, DC 20001, Jan./Feb.

Chilman, C. S. (1980). Social and psychological research concerning adolescent childbearing: 1970–1980. *Journal of Marriage and the Family, 42*, 793–805.

Epstein, M. F. (1979). Children living in one parent families. *Monthly Labor News, 102*, 21–32.

Forrest, J. D., & Singh, S. (1990). The sexual and reproductive behavior of American women, 1982–1988. *Family Planning Perspectives, 22*, 206–214.

Furstenberg, F. F. (1987). Race differences in teenage sexuality, pregnancy and adolescent childbearing, *Millbank Q, 65* (Suppl. 2), 381–403.

Furstenberg, F. F., & Crawford, A. G. (1978). Family support: Helping teenage mothers to cope. *Family Planning Perspective, 15*, 322–333.

Franklin, D. (1988). Race, class and adolescent pregnancy: An ecological analysis. *American Journal of Orthopsychiatry, 58*, 339–351.

Hatcher, R. A., Stewart, F., Trussell, J., Kowal, D., Quest, F., Stewart, G., & Cates, W. (1990). *Contraceptive technology: 1990–1992* (15th rev. ed.) New York: Irvington.

Henshaw, S. K., & Van Vort, J. (Eds.). (1990). Teenage abortion, birth and pregnancy statistics: An update. *Family Planning Perspectives, 21*, 85–88.

Hofferth, S., Kahn, J., & Baldwin, W. (1987). Premarital sexual activity among U.S. teenagers over the past three decades. *Family Planning Perspectives, 19*, 46–53.

Hofferth, S. L., & Moore, K. A. (1979). Early childbearing and later economic well being. *American Sociological Review, 44*, 784–815.

Hogan, D., & Kitagawa, E. (1985). The impact of social status, family structure and neighborhood on the fertility of Black adolescents. *American Journal of Sociology, 90*, 825–853.

Johnson, R. E., Namias, A., Magder, L. S., Lee, F., Brooks, C., & Snowden, C. (1989). A seroepidemiologic survey of the prevalence of herpes simplex virus type 2 in the United States. *New England Journal of Medicine, 321,* 7–12.

Lewis, O. (1966). *La vida.* New York: Random House.

Mosher, W. (1990). Contraceptive practice in the United States, 1982–1988. *Family Planning Perspective, 22,* 198–205.

National Center for Health Statistics. (1990). Contraceptive use in the United States, 1973–1988. *Advance data from Vital and Health Statistics of the National Center for Health Statistics, 182.*

Pittman, K., & Adams, G. (1988). Teenage pregnancy: An advocate's guide to the numbers. Washington, DC: Children's Defense Fund.

Pratt, W. F., Mosher W., Bachrach, C., & Harn, M. (1984). Understanding U.S. fertility: Findings from the National Survey of Family Growth: Cycle III *Population Bulletin, 39,* 1–42.

Rainwater, L., & Yancy, W. L. (1967). *The Moynihan report and the politics of controversy.* Cambridge, MA: MIT Press.

Reid, J. (1982). Black America in the 1980s. *Population Bulletin, 37,* 1–39.

Rhodes, M. L. (1992). *Contraceptive behavior of adolescent females aged 12–18.* Manuscript submitted for publication.

Stack, C. (1974). Sex roles and survival strategies in the urban black community. In M. Zimbaliso-Rosaldo & L. Lamphere (Eds.), *Culture and society* (pp. 113–28). Stanford, CA: Stanford University Press.

Staples, R. (1973). *Adolescent sexuality in contemporary America.* New York: World Publishers.

Trussell, J. (1988). Teenage pregnancy in the United States. *Family Planning Perspectives, 20,* 262–271.

U.S. Bureau of the Census. (1985). Money, income and poverty status of families and persons in the United States: 1984 (Advanced Report). *Current Population Reports,* (Series P–60, No. 149). Washington, DC: U.S. Government Printing Office.

U.S. Bureau of the Census. (1990). *Statistical abstract of the United States: 1990* (110th ed.) Washington, DC: U.S. Government Printing Office.

U. S. Bureau of the Census. *Statistical abstract of the United States: 1992* (112th ed.). Washington DC: U.S. Government Printing Office.

U.S. Department of Commerce, Bureau of the Census. (1983). Population profile of the United States: 1982. *Current population reports* (Special Studies Series P–23, No. 103). Washington, DC: U.S. Government Printing Office.

Westoff, C. F. (1988). Unintended pregnancy in America and abroad. *Family Planning Perspectives, 20,* 254–261.

Wetzel, J. R. (1987). American youth: A statistical snapshot. Washington, DC: William T. Grant Foundation.

Zabin, L., Hirsch, M., Smith, E., Emerson, M., King, T., Street, R., & Hardy, J. (1988). The Baltimore pregnancy prevention program for urban teenagers: What did it cost? *Family Planning Perspectives, 20,* 188–192.

Zelnik, M., & Kantner, J. F. (1977). Sexual and contraceptive experiences of young unmarried women in the United States, 1966–1971. *Family Planning Perspectives, 9,* 55–73.

Zelnik, M., Kantner, J. F., & Ford, K. (1981). *Sex and pregnancy in adolescence.* Beverly Hills, CA: Sage.

9

Ethical and Legal Controversies in Critical Care Nursing

Yvonne K. Scherer and Michael H. Ackerman

Intensive care units (ICUs) and the specialty of critical care nursing that began with them have come a long way since they were introduced into the health care system in the late 1950s and early 1960s. Today there are coronary care units (CCUs), surgical intensive care units (SICUs), medical intensive care units (MICUs), trauma units, and others. These units are highly specialized to meet the acute care needs of the patients admitted into them. These specialized units contain very sophisticated equipment designed to monitor and sustain life. Mechanical ventilators breathe for those who cannot, ventricular assist devices support a failing heart, and hemodialysis machines take over the function of diseased kidneys. If individuals die, cardiopulmonary resuscitation can bring them back to life. Diseased organs can be replaced by organs transplanted from another individual. Individuals can receive new hearts, new kidneys, new livers, and new lungs. The ability to sustain life has reached new limits. While this is a remarkable accomplishment, it does pose problems. Death is no longer a natural phenomenon over which we have no control.

The critical care nurse, in addition to becoming adept at carrying out very sophisticated procedures, must grapple with the many legal and ethical questions that this highly technological environment has created. Two of the most common issues center in "Do Not Resuscitate" orders and transplantation. These two particular areas will be explored in detail, as they are areas where the nurse is able to make an optimal contribution for the patient as well as the family.

CARDIOPULMONARY RESUSCITATION (CPR)

CPR is the restoration of heartbeat and/or breathing through medical intervention. Basic resuscitation involves the maintenance of respiration and heartbeat through artificial resuscitation and external chest compression. Advanced resuscitation involves more sophisticated techniques, such as the use of a defibrillator to shock the heart and stimulate cardiac contractions. Unless cardiac and respiratory function are restored within 4–5 minutes of arrest, irreversible brain damage and death will occur. CPR is the presumed course of action in cases of cardiac and respiratory failure in acute care settings.

The results of CPR may be successful or unsuccessful. If successful, the patient may assume a normal way of life, if unsuccessful, the patient will die. Partial success may leave the patient brain-damaged or too debilitated to ever leave the hospital.

Since CPR must be applied rapidly to be effective, there frequently is not time to consider the appropriateness of the action. When CPR was introduced in the 1960s, most physicians felt obligated to use this technology for all patients. Yet several studies have shown that CPR has been effective only in a small minority of hospitalized patients (Luce & Raffin, 1988). Approximately one out of three patients are resuscitated with CPR. Of patients who are resuscitated approximately 3% to 30% are discharged from the hospital. Lower success rates occur in patients with severe diseases, such as chronic obstructive lung disease (Bedell, 1984). In order to prevent the indiscriminate use of CPR, the American Heart Association advocated that CPR need not be used in patients with terminal, irreversible illness whose death is expected and in whom resuscitation represents a violation of the right to die with dignity (American Heart Association, 1986).

DO NOT RESUSCITATE (DNR) ORDERS

A DNR order in a patient's chart basically means that CPR measures will be withheld in the event of a cardiac or respiratory arrest (Miles, Cranford, & Schultz, 1982). DNR orders have created many ethical dilemmas for health care professionals today. These dilemmas become even more complex when DNR orders are written for patients in ICUs. The emergence of DNR orders resulted from the growing recognition that resuscitation was neither medically appropriate for nor consistent with the wishes of all patients. As experience with CPR increased, it became evident that for certain patients it offered only a more violent death.

Problems Arising from the Use of DNR Orders

Two problems have occurred as the result of DNR orders. The first is the writing of DNR orders without the consent of patients or their family members. The second is the resuscitation of patients in circumstances where resuscitation is not medically indicated (New York State Task Force on Life and the Law, 1988).

The use of DNR orders without consent is not as problematic as it once was. In the past, a colored dot was placed on a patient's chart to signify a DNR. This negated the need to put a written DNR order in the patient's chart. This system was devised in response to the idea that DNR orders were of doubtful legality. The use of "slow code" and the "show code" were also instituted in hospitals. In a "slow code", resuscitation efforts were carried out in a manner designed to fail, such as taking more time calling the resuscitation team to the patient's bedside. A "show code" was activity carried out for the benefit of the patient's family to make it appear that resuscitation is being carried out (New York State Task Force on Life and the Law, 1988). Both "slow" and "show" codes were aimed at only going through the motions of CPR without actually instituting any resuscitative measures.

The dot system, slow code, and show code were all measures designed to achieve the results of a DNR order without risking any legal liability. The courts did not sanction these covert methods of issuing DNR orders, and these measures were considered to be unethical and illicit.

The second problem associated with CPR is the resuscitation of patients when it is not medically appropriate since the resuscitation will probably fail. Resuscitation of patients when not medically indicated can be especially problematic in the ICU setting. Patients are acutely ill and it is somewhat expected that every effort will be instituted to maintain life. There are also other reasons why CPR may be carried out on medically inappropriate patients. Physicians may feel uncomfortable in carrying on discussions about DNR orders with competent patients and their families. Factors such as the physician's personal fear of death, guilt over being unable to save the patient, insecurity in dealing with highly emotional, value-laden issues, and a sense of failure have all been cited as reasons for physicians having difficulty in discussing the DNR order with patients (Miller & Lo, 1985; Ruark & Raffin, 1988). In one study (Stolman, Gregory, Dunn, & Levine, 1990) it was found that 30% of the 60 physicians interviewed said they were uncomfortable discussing resuscitation with the patient. Furthermore, patients in the ICU are usually cared for by a team of physicians rather than one doctor. This can cause difficulties in coming to a consensus about the initiation of a DNR order. In addition, physicians and other members of the health care team many times hold on to the belief that this may be the one miraculous patient that is saved through their medical interventions.

Lack of nurse involvement in the resuscitation issue may also contribute to failure to obtain an appropriate DNR order. Although responsibility for the DNR order resides in the physician-patient interaction, nurses can be of assistance in facilitating the process. Nurses' noninvolvement in the DNR process may be due in part to the current nursing shortage, that allows less time with each patient and family. It may also be due to a reluctance on the nurse's part to assume a responsibility which has traditionally been the physician's, and the fear of repercussions from physicians if nurses become involved in the resuscitation issue. However, the nurse must actively collaborate with the physician, patient and/or family in the decisionmaking process regarding DNR. Stolman et al. (1990) found that the 77 nurses interviewed were not often involved in discussion of resuscitation decisions with patients or families. Conversely, the study reported that informal discussions with nursing staff revealed that nurses were sensitive to resuscitation issues and were often the ones who alerted the physicians to the patients' and families' wishes regarding resuscitation.

Resuscitation of patients when not medically indicated may occur because critically ill patients tend to suffer from unanticipated problems such as stroke, trauma, or postoperative complications. These complications often have occurred before patients have expressed their wishes regarding treatment (Luce & Raffin, 1988). Not knowing a patient's wishes regarding a DNR order can make it difficult for physicians and families to reach a decision.

Finally, family members may demand aggressive treatment regardless of the benefits or burdens it causes for the patient. Family members may be unwilling to accept the fact that the patient is dying or they may be unable to resolve guilt feelings about allowing the patient to die. Also, conflict among family members regarding the appropriateness of DNR orders can cause delays resulting in the initiation of resuscitative measures.

Values Underlying Resuscitation Decisions

Advances in medical technology can help to preserve life. However, individuals should have the right to choose whether or not that technology is appropriate for them. The dignity of each person requires a deep respect for the freedom and autonomy of individuals to make decisions about their own lives.

Autonomy has special significance with regard to CPR. The benefit of prolonging a life which could potentially be filled with suffering and disability must be weighed against the possibility of an earlier more peaceful and dignified death. Respect for autonomy recognizes the patient's right to request or refuse CPR. Although adherence to patient autonomy is important, especially for those who are acutely ill, patients are frequently overwhelmed by their illness and welcome decisionmaking assistance from families, physicians, and nurses.

According to Stolman et al. (1990) the majority of the 97 patients interviewed in their study did not think discussing the hypothetical topic of resuscitation was cruel and insensitive. Patients gave a variety of reasons for not wanting to be resuscitated. About half of the reasons were related to "quality-of-life" issues such as "I don't want to be a burden or a vegetable" and "I'm tired of living." The researchers also found that most of the patients (66%) preferred shared decisionmaking and that if there was a disagreement many (41%) wanted their views to be decisive. Few patients opted for noninvolvement in decision making.

There is a high rate of morbidity and mortality and a large number of invasive procedures carried out in the ICU because of the seriousness and complexity of the diseases seen in patients who are admitted to the unit. Therefore, it would seem appropriate to discuss preferences concerning aggressive care such as CPR with these patients. Blackhall, Cobb, and Moskowitz (1989) carried out a 9-month study on 611 patients admitted to ICUs to determine how frequently the issue of resuscitation was discussed with the patients. They found that only 11% of patients or their families were involved in discussions regarding the appropriateness of aggressive care. These findings are consistent with those of other studies (Bedell & Delbanco, 1984; Evans & Brody, 1985). These findings also showed that such discussions occurred more frequently with those patients who were elderly, demented, or had a poor prognosis or a high acuity level. Zimmerman, Knaus, Sharpe, Anderson, Draper, & Wagner (1986) reported similar findings.

The fact that studies indicate that only small numbers of acutely ill patients and/or their families are approached concerning DNR is distressing. This is especially so in that physicians have been shown to differ significantly from their patients in assessing quality of life. In addition, physicians are unable to predict their patients' preferences regarding resuscitation (Evans & Brody, 1985; Starr, Pearlman, & Uhlman, 1986).

Discrepancies have also been shown between physicians and patients as to their perceptions of having discussed resuscitation. The use of medical jargon, communicating through third parties, informing a little at a time, and communicating in an indirect manner can affect patient understanding, perception, and recollection of physician discussion of the DNR order (Stolman et al., 1990).

The Noncompetent Patient

As the patient's competency to make decisions diminishes, the family's role in decisionmaking increases. Family members are considered to be most knowledgeable of the preferences and wishes of the patient and are best able to protect those interests. This is particularly true when it is a child who is ill. Parental autonomy in such matters is usually recognized by the state (New York State Task Force on Life and the Law, 1988).

When adults lack the capacity to make decisions concerning their medical care, the question arises as to who—family, another person, the state—should be given the power to make decisions on their behalf. Perhaps the best known judicial decision regarding withholding and withdrawal of life support took place in the case of Karen Quinlan in 1975. The 22-year-old woman was in a persistent vegetative state and her father petitioned the court to appoint him her guardian with the power to remove her from mechanical ventilation. The court ruled in favor of the father's petition, stating that patients generally would accept or refuse medical treatment based on its ability to support sentient life as distinguished from mere biologic existence. The court concluded that Karen Quinlan would have decided to forgo life-prolonging therapy if she was not in a vegetative state. The court therefore granted the father "substituted judgement" for his daughter (Luce & Raffin, 1988).

There were other court cases that upheld the concept of "substituted judgement," one of which specifically related to the DNR order. In "The Matter of Dinnerstein" (1978), the court supported the family of a 67-year-old woman with Alzheimer's disease who had petitioned the court for a judgement that a DNR order could be written in her medical record without judicial approval. In Barber vs. Superior Court (1983) the court held that, without evidence of malevolence, family members are the proper surrogates for an incompetent patient, and that prior judicial approval is not necessary if families and physicians decide to withhold or withdraw support (Luce & Raffin, 1988).

The courts have also endorsed the use of patients' previously stated wishes regarding life support. These wishes can be expressed in a living will, a document that contains a person's instructions about treatment to be followed in the event that they become incapable of making treatment decisions on their own. The directives set down in a living will can provide valuable guidance to family members and health care providers. Problems do exist with living wills in that the application of the written document to a particular situation may be unclear. A decision expressed in a living will to forego "extraordinary measures" may not apply in every situation. For example, CPR may not be an "extraordinary measure" to apply to an otherwise healthy person who has suffered a heart attack (New York State Task Force on Life and the Law, 1988).

Another, perhaps more useful directive is the Health Care Proxy document, that empowers competent adults to appoint an agent to decide about health care in the event they become unable to decide. The health care agent can be any competent adult. Certain persons may for themselves be excluded, as health care agents and these individuals are identified in state guidelines. The appointment of a health care agent avoids the difficulty, inherent in the use of living wills, of trying to anticipate future medical care needs. The agent's decisionmaking authority begins when the patient's physician, using set criteria, determines that the patient lacks the capacity to decide about health care (New York State Task Force on Life and the Law, 1987). The Health Care Proxy is considered a legal document in most states and each state provides specific guidelines for its use. The Proxy avoids the threat of liability in withholding CPR in an incompetent patient whose wishes regarding life sustaining treatment are unknown. Such a document may also avoid disagreements that may arise among family members regarding a DNR order.

The DNR Order

The directives for a DNR order may vary somewhat from state to state, but the basic components of the order are similar. To enter a DNR order for competent patients, the patient, unless it is deemed unadvisable by the physician, must be informed about his/her condition, risks/benefits of CPR, and consequences of the DNR order. Oral or written consent must be obtained from the patient. The patient's decision and the DNR order are recorded in the chart. The same protocol is followed with incompetent patients except that a surrogate or health care agent makes the decision. In patients who lack capacity or have no surrogate, the decision for a DNR order is made by at least two physicians. Considerations need to be made for competent patients who for one reason or another do not want discussion of or involvement in resuscitation decisions. Discussion of a DNR order may be upsetting or even harmful to them. To help patients who may fall into this category, hospital DNR policies should provide a method for writing DNR orders without direct patient consent. The use of a surrogate decisionmaker empowered to make a "substituted judgement" may be one way to deal with this issue (Stolman et al., 1990).

Once the DNR order has been written, it often becomes necessary to make decisions about which specific treatments should be initiated, withheld, or discontinued with DNR patients. This is especially appropriate in the ICU, where advanced lifesaving technology is commonplace. At one extreme is the belief that, with the exception of cardiopulmonary resuscitation, all medical interventions should be continued and/or initiated for DNR patients. At the other extreme is the belief that DNR patients should be allowed to die quietly and with dignity. In the latter case there would be limitations of treatment and some or all life-sustaining medical interventions would be withdrawn and only the use of comfort measures would be employed (Lewandowski, Daly, McClish, Tuknialis, & Younger, 1985).

Another major issue is whether the use of costly ICU resources for DNR patients can be justified. Findings from a study by Lewandowski et al. (1985) of patients admitted to a medical intensive care unit indicated that a DNR order is neither an indication that physicians and nurses will cease to care for the patients, nor a mandate for transfer out of the ICU. The study found that DNR patients consumed enormous amounts of ICU resources. The DNR order had a limited influence on the withdrawal of specific aggressive therapies such as medications and use of ventilators. The DNR order also did not influence the amount of nursing care directed toward meeting the physical needs of patients.

DNR Issues

Many issues are involved in the DNR decision in the acute care setting. Initially, formal policies for DNR orders must be written. In order to meet the goal of decisionmaking before a crisis, methods need to be developed to overcome reluctance by medical personnel to discuss the DNR order with patients and/or families. This will help to ensure that the patients, or those closest to them, will retain the autonomy to make this important decision. Many feel that the discussion regarding DNR should take place on admission to the hospital. Critical care nurses need to assist patients and their families with the DNR process. Critical care nurses spend anywhere from 8 to 13 hours a day with patients and their families. This puts them in an ideal situation to assess patients' and families' wishes regarding the DNR order. The nurse therefore has a unique opportunity to act as facilitator between patients, family, and physician in arriving at a DNR decision.

Critical care nurses must make sure that their personal feelings regarding DNR orders do not influence their relationships with patients and families whose beliefs may differ from their own. Each individual's view of quality of life needs to be respected. The nurse's role is to listen, provide emotional support, and to reassure patients and families that they will be given proper care. The wishes of informed patients and/or family members regarding a DNR order need to be respected.

As a result of the confusion and the gray areas associated with DNR issues, and to give patients a large degree of autonomy, the Patient Self-Determination Act (PSDA) was passed into law. This act is part of the Omnibus Reconciliation Act of 1990 and was put into force in December, 1991. Along with the PSDA is the recognition of the need for advanced directives such as Living Wills and Power of Attorney for Health Care (Flarey, 1991). The PSDA has essentially five requirements (Hassmiller, 1991). Upon admission to the hospital, patients are asked whether or not they have an advanced directive and are given information concerning the hospital policies on advanced directives; hospitals must document whether or not the patient has an advanced directive in the medical record; discrimination must be prohibited based on whether or not the patient has an advanced directive; and the hospital must provide staff and community education concerning the PSDA.

The Health Care Financing Administration has been charged with overseeing that hospitals comply with the regulations of the PSDA (Wolf, et al., 1991). Hospitals that do not comply may get less or even lose Medicaid and Medicare funding. To date there have been many issues regarding the implementation of this Act. Danis and colleagues (1991) in a prospective study found that the care administered to patients in one nursing home and one hospital was consistent with the patient's previously expressed wishes only 75% of the time. The fact that the advanced directive was present in the medical record did not increase the likelihood that the patient's wishes would be adhered to. One of the conclusions of this study was that better enforcement mechanisms must be developed in this area, in order to optimally implement advanced directives as well as allow patients the autonomy that they deserve. Emanuel, Barry, Stoeckle, Ettelson, and Emmanuel (1991) found that the most frequent barrier to issuing an advanced directive was not the fact that it is such a sensitive issue, but the physician's failure to initiate the topic. The conception that patients will not want to address the advanced directive because of its sensitivity is a common misconception; with further research in this area, more of these misconceptions can be eliminated.

ORGAN AND TISSUE TRANSPLANTATION

Improved technology, immunosuppressive therapy, and an improvement in insurance funding have led to an increased demand for organs for transplantation. Although efforts have been made to increase the number of organs available, the supply cannot keep pace with the demand. Those ethical and legal issues surrounding transplantation that have the greatest impact on nurses who work in acute care settings are related to organ procurement, recipient candidacy, and allocation of health care resources.

Historical Perspective

The first successful organ transplantation occurred in 1953, when a kidney from a living, related donor was successfully transplanted. Studies of the immune system and methods of controlling rejection began between 1955 and 1962. The introduction of azathioprine coupled with prednisone dramatically increased graft survival and began the era of transplantation. The FDA approval of cyclosporine, a potent immuno-suppressive agent, for general use in the United States in 1983 greatly helped to reduce rejection of transplanted organs. As a result of these medical advances, the demand for organs such as the kidney, heart, and liver now greatly exceeds the supply (Palumbi, 1990).

To accommodate the increase in demand for organs, laws and organizational procedures to improve the procurement process have been developed and implemented over the past 30 years. The Uniform Anatomical Gift Act (UAGA) which was adapted by all 50 states in 1973 served as a model for states whose laws did not clearly define a person's ability to donate his or her organs. The act fostered organ donation by providing: 1) a legal framework for the use of donor cards, 2) physician protection from legal complications of organ donation, and 3) civil and criminal protection for persons acting in good faith and in compliance with guidelines while participating in the procurement process (Rivers et al., 1990a).

In 1978 the United Network of Organ Sharing (UNOS) established a computer system to match patients in need of transplants with donor centers. Additional functions were assigned to UNOS in 1986. These included the development of standards for procurement and transplantation and the establishment of a board of directors whose main responsibility was to guarantee equitable sharing of organs. Passage of the Omnibus Budget Reconciliation Act in 1986 required written protocols for donor identification and referral to hospitals participating in Medicare-Medicaid programs. In 1988, the Required Request laws were adopted by 43 states. These laws require hospitals to develop guidelines so that families have the right to choose between voluntary donation and refusal (Rivers et al., 1990b). Despite these legal and organizational undertakings, a chronic shortage of organs for transplantation still exists. This shortage has prompted individuals to consider other measures to improve the supply of these organs.

Controversial Issues in Organ Procurement

Some controversial measures which have been proposed to assist in alleviating the organ shortage problem include redefining the definition of brain death, use of anencephalic newborns, xenografts, and presumed consent.

Redefining the Definition of Brain Death

The advent of sophisticated equipment such as respiratory ventilators, which keep individuals alive regardless of their brain activity caused the medical profession to take a closer look at the definition of death. In 1968 an ad hoc committee of the Harvard Medical School established guidelines for the diagnosis of cerebral death based on cessation of neurologic function (Grenvik, 1988). In 1980, due to a lack of uniformity of statutes on brain death, members of the President's Commission for the Study of Ethical Problems in Medicine and Biomedical and Behavioral Research developed a uniform model law referred to as the Uniform Determination of Death Act. This Act provided a comprehensive basis for determining death in all situations. All 50 states have either adopted a form of the Uniform Determination of Death Act or had precedent set in appellate court decisions (Neely & Davis, 1990). Basically, brain death is medically defined as the irreversible cessation of all brain activity, which means that both the cerebrum and brain stem have ceased to function. There are those who argue that the definition of brain death should not include the cessation of brain stem activity. These individuals endorse a concept of death based on attributes largely associated with the cerebrum (higher brain concept), such as consciousness and cognition (Younger, Landefeld, Coulton, Tuknialis, & Leary, 1989). The brain stem controls basic functions such as respiration and general body movement. Acceptance of the higher brain concept would permit organ retrieval from patients in a persistent vegetative coma as well as from anencephalic newborns. Ethical issues which need to be considered in defining brain death center around what constitutes human life. Also public fear that death would be hastened to get organs for transplantation could be greatly exacerbated (Rivers et al., 1990b).

Anencephalic Newborns

Presently organs for transplantation are obtained from heart-beating cadavers that lack all brain function including the brain stem. However, the increasing demand for pediatric organs has focused attention on obtaining these organs from anencephalic newborns. These infants have a functioning brain stem, but no cerebrum: These babies can maintain vital functions such as heartbeat and respiration from several hours to several days, but eventually develop respiratory failure and die. Those who advocate defining brain death at the cortical level argue that vital organs could be harvested from these infants who are going to die anyway. These people believe that these infants can save other lives, thereby benefiting the recipient, the parents of the recipient, and the parents of the donor. Conversely, those who accept the legal and medical definition of brain death argue that this would be an infringement on the personhood of the infant as well as raising issues of respect and dignity (Rothenberg, 1990).

Xenografts

Another controversial issue involves the use of xenografts, or animal organs, to combat the organ shortage. Early attempts at the transplantation of xenografts were unsuccessful. This procedure was again carried out in 1984 when "Baby Fae" received the heart of a baboon. More recently, in 1992, a baboon liver was transplanted into a human with much resulting controversy. Ethical dilemmas arise over the experimental nature of the procedure and infringement of animal rights (Rivers et al., 1990a).

Presumed Consent

The concept of presumed consent would give health care professionals the authority to remove organs from cadavers for transplantation. The consent of the deceased and the family to donation is assumed unless they have objected. Consent is not solicited; rather, the objections of the family or those of the deceased must be conveyed in an explicit manner. Those who advocate this policy view organs and tissues as a community resource that should be used to benefit society. Those opposed to this policy believe that it infringes on an individual's autonomy, respect, and dignity (Rivers et al., 1990a, 1990b). In countries where such a law exists, physicians continue to seek permission from family members and do not remove organs if families object (Marsden, 1988).

Other proposals to improve the supply of organs include a free market system allowing individuals to buy or sell organs; income and estate tax credits; and routine referral to organ procurement agencies of admissions that are likely to lead to organ donation situations (Rivers et al., 1990). Although some advocate a more aggressive approach to increasing the amount of transplantable organs, voluntarism and informed consent have been the underlying values structuring the organ donation policy in this country (Marsden, 1988).

Critical care nurses need to be clear regarding their role and responsibilities in organ transplantation. Nurses need to be knowledgeable regarding suitable donors and how to notify the appropriate people. They also need to explore their own feelings and beliefs regarding organ procurement. Some nurses may find it difficult to approach a family member about organ donation, others may believe that organ donation is morally wrong. Institutional policies need to be in place to help nurses deal with their concerns regarding organ procurement.

Specific nursing responsibilities involved in caring for transplantation will vary according to state as well as by institution. These responsibilities can be divided into two areas: donor care and recipient care. Recipient care will depend upon the organ or tissue transplanted. Most transplant recipients will require post-transplant care in a critical care unit for close observation and monitoring. Nursing responsibilities for transplant donors can include identification of potential donors, approaching family members about possible organ donation, notification of organ procurement officials, and maintaining a patient for organ harvesting. Many institutions have specific individuals responsible for approaching family members and notification of organ procurement agencies; however, others may not and the responsibility may fall on the critical care nurse.

In a study by Stoeckle (1990), 44 critical care nurses' attitudes toward organ donation were assessed. Ninety-five percent indicated a positive to strongly positive attitude toward the concept of organ donation. Analysis of knowledge levels indicated that the nurses demonstrated a lack of knowledge of the organ donor identification and management criteria. The study showed that nurses benefit from the experience of providing care for organ donors, recipients, and their families, and that increased knowledge about organ procurement was correlated with improved attitudes. Providing support for the family of an organ donor was reported as being emotionally draining by 71% of the nurses. The researcher concluded that educational programs in the area of organ donor identification and management are necessary and that emotional support needs to be provided to these nurses. Comparable findings were reported by Bidigare and Oermann (1991). More research is needed in the area of organ procurement and its effects on nurses' attitudes and their care of donors as well as recipients.

Recipient Candidacy

A second issue surrounding the ethical dilemma of organ transplantation is recipient selection. Since not enough transplantable organs are available, decisions regarding who will and who will not receive them pose many ethical problems. Controversies arise over who should make the final decision and what criteria for candidate selection is appropriate. For example, should criteria such as the candidate's age, character, and accomplishments be factors? Equity is a critical issue. Are multiple transplants in one patient justified? Donated organs must be distributed fairly, without discrimination or bias, and in a way that produces the greatest good to humanity (Neely & Davis, 1990).

Patient selection is divided into three phases. The first phase deals with objective medical data which confirms the need and suitability of the recipient. A financial assessment is also conducted to determine if the patient has private insurance to assist with medical expenses. If the patient has no private insurance, an assessment is done to determine who will pay for the transplant procedure. Phase II deals with subjective criteria; for example, will the patient be compliant with the follow-up regimen? Psychiatric evaluations of patients and families may be carried out. Those patients meeting the criteria in phases I and II are pooled. In Phase III, decisions must be made as to whom in this pool receives an organ as it becomes available. The Organ Procurement Transplant Network has significantly standardized this process and have attempted to develop criteria that are fair (Neely & Davis, 1990).

Despite efforts to maintain fairness in organ transplantation, problems do exist. The danger exists that transplantations will become a product for the white upper and middle classes. These individuals are more likely to have good compliance records and stable support systems. Efforts need to be directed toward developing criteria that are independent of social worth categories. Also, questions arise as to when the obligation to do all that is possible prolongs death instead of life (Marsden, 1988).

Allocation of Health Care Resources

Another ethical issue which arises in organ transplantation is the question of whether the government should provide wider societal access to organ transplantation which would likely limit access to other kinds of health care. The Health Care Financing Administration (HCFA), which administers Medicare, has investigated the allocation of health care dollars for transplantation. This is due in part to the government's experience with the extraordinarily high cost of providing universal entitlement for kidney transplant. However, even with limited funding, approval for transplantation by Medicare will only benefit those individuals with a work history who have been disabled for two years or for those over 65 years of age, and therefore only a limited population (Marsden, 1988). The question then arises as to whether or not Medicare dollars should be reallocated to defray the costs of a procedure that will benefit only a minority of the population it serves. Should valuable health care dollars be spent on organ transplants, or on preventative health care instead?

The President's Commission for the Study of Ethical Problems in Medicine and Biomedical and Behavioral Research concluded that society has an ethical obligation to insure equal access to an adequate level of health care for all (President's Commission for the Study of Ethical Problems in Medicine and Behavioral Research, 1983). Does providing some forms of health care, such as expensive organ transplantation, endanger equal access to an adequate level of health care for all? Society needs to take a careful look at the distribution of health care and its impact on a person's well-being (Marsden, 1988).

Nurses need to be cognizant of health care legislation and the impact of this legislation on health promotion, disease prevention, and treatment. Whenever possible, nurses need to make legislatures aware of important health care issues such as organ transplantation and lobby for legislation that aims at a fair distribution of health care for all. In addition, more research needs to be carried out that looks at the effect of procedures such as organ transplantation on quality of life.

CONCLUSION AND TOPICS FOR DISCUSSION

Technology has forced us to deal with the issues of DNR and organ transplantation. Nurses in the acute care setting need to be cognizant of the moral and ethical considerations involved in the formation of policy concerning these issues. Nurses must strive to maintain the highest regard for human dignity and quality of life while supporting the technological and scientific advances of our society. The following are topics for discussion:

TOPICS FOR DISCUSSION

1. Should CPR be initiated on a terminally ill patient?
2. Should terminally ill patients be admitted to the ICU?
3. How involved should the critical care nurse become in the DNR process?
4. How might you intervene in a situation where there is a controversy between the family and physician regarding the initiating of a DNR order?
5. Analyze your own feelings regarding DNR orders.
6. How do you feel about animal organs being transplanted into humans?
7. How do you feel about limiting transplantation only to those who have the financial resources to pay for the transplant?
8. Do you feel that more federal health care dollars should go into disease prevention, or into transplantation?
9. How do you feel about the current definition of "brain death"?
10. Have you designated yourself as an organ donor?

REFERENCES

American Health Association. (1986). Standards and guidelines for cardiopulmonary resuscitation and emergency cardiac care. *Journal of the American Medical Association, 255,* 2841–3044.

Bedell, S. (1984). Long-term survival after pre-hospital sudden cardiac death. *American Heart Journal, 108,* 1–4.

Bedell, S. E., & Delbanco, T. L. (1984). Choices about cardiopulmonary resuscitation in the hospital: When do physicians talk with patients? *New England Journal of Medicine, 310,* 1089–1093.

Bidigare, S. A., & Oermann, M. H. (1991). Attitudes and knowledge of nurses regarding organ procurement. *Organ Transplantation, 20,* 20–24.

Blackhall, L. T., Cobb, T., & Moskowitz, M. A. (1989). Discussions regarding aggressive care with critically ill patients. *Journal of General Internal Medicine, 4,* 399–402.

Danis, M., Southerland, L. J., Garrett, J. M., Smith J. L., Hielema, F., Pickard C. G., Egnar, D. M., & Patrick, D. L. (1991). A prospective study of advance directives for life sustaining care. *New England Journal of Medicine, 324,* 882–888.

Emanuel, L. L., Barry, M. J., Stoeckle, J. D., Ettleson, L. M., & Emmanuel, E. J. (1991). Advance directives for medical care: A case for greater use. *New England Journal of Medicine, 324,* 889–895.

Evans, A. L. & Brody, B. A. (1985). The do-not-resuscitate order in teaching hospitals. *Journal of the American Medical Association, 253,* 2236–2239.

Flarey, D. L. (1991). Advanced directives: In search of self-determination. *Journal of Nursing Administration, 21,* 16–22.

Grenvik, A. (1988). Ethical dilemmas in organ donation and transplantation. *Critical Care Medicine, 16,* 1012–1018.

Hassmiller, S. (1991). Bringing the patient self-determination act into practice. *Nursing Management, 22,* 27–32.

Lewandowski, W., Daly, B., McClish, D., Tuknialis, B., & Younger, S. T. (1985). Treatment and care of "do not resuscitate" patients in a medical intensive care unit. *Heart & Lung, 14,* 175–181.

Luce, T. M. & Raffin, T. A. (1988). Withholding and withdrawal of life support from critically ill patients. *Chest, 94,* 621–626.

Marsden, C. (1988). Ethical issues in cardiac transplantation. *Journal of Cardiovascular Nursing, 2,* 23–30.

Miles, S. H., Cranford, R., & Schultz, A. L. (1982). The do-not-resuscitate order in a teaching hospital. *Annals of Internal Medicine, 96,* 660–665.

Miller, A., & Lo, B. (1985). How do doctors discuss do-not-resuscitate orders? *Western Journal of Medicine, 143,* 256–258.

Neely, S., & Davis, N. S. (1990). Legal and ethical issues. In K. M. Sigardson-Poor & C. R. Haggerty (Eds.), *Nursing care of the transplant recipient* (pp. 395–421). Philadelphia: Saunders Company.

New York State Task Force on Life and the Law. (1987). *Life-sustaining treatment: Making decisions and appointing a health care agent.* New York State.

New York State Task Force on Life and the Law. (1988). *Do-not-resuscitate orders: The proposed legislation and report of the New York State Task Force on Life and the Law.* New York State.

Palumbi, M. A. (1990). Historical perspective. In Sigardson-Poor & Haggerty (Eds.), *Nursing care of the transplant recipient* (pp. 1–11). Philadelphia: Saunders.

President's Commission for the Study of Ethical Problems in Medicine and Behavioral Research. (1983). *Securing access to health care.* Washington, DC: U.S. Government Printing Office.

Rivers, E. P., Buse, S. M., Bivins, B. A., & Horst, H. M. (1990a). Organ and tissue procurement in the acute care setting: Principles and practice: Part I. *Annals of Emergency Medicine, 19,* 78–85.

Rivers, E. P., Buse, S. M., Bivins, B. A., & Horst, H. M. (1990b). Organ and tissue procurement in the acute care setting: Principles and practice: Part II. *Annals of Emergency Medicine, 19*, 193–200.

Rothenberg, L. S. (1990). The anencephalic neonate and brain death: An international review of medical, ethical, and legal issues. *Transplantation Proceedings, 22*, 1037–1039.

Ruark, T. E. & Raffin, T .A. (1988). Initiating and withdrawing life support: Principles and practices in adult medicine. *New England Journal of Medicine, 318*, 25–30.

Starr, T. J., Pearlman, R. A., & Uhlman, R. F. (1986). Quality of life and resuscitation decisions in elderly patients. *Journal of General Internal Medicine, 1*, 373–379.

Stoeckle, M. L. (1990). Attitudes of critical care nurses toward organ donation. *Dimensions of Critical Care Nursing, 9*, 354–361.

Stolman, C. T., Gregory, T. T., Dunn, D., & Levine, T. T. (1990). Evaluation of patient, physician, nurse, and family attitudes toward do-not-resuscitate orders. *Archives of Internal Medicine, 150*, 653–658.

Wolf, S. M., Boyle, P., Callahan, D., Fins, J. J., Jennings, B., Nelson, J. L., Barondess, J. A., Brock, D. W., Dresser, R., & Emmanuel, L. (1991). Sources of concern about the Patient Self-Determination Act. *New England Journal of Medicine, 325*, 1666–1671.

Younger, S. T., Landefeld, S., Coulton, C. T., Tukialis, B. W., & Leary, M. (1989). Brain death and organ retrieval: A cross-sectional survey of knowledge and concepts among health professionals. *Journal of the American Medical Association, 261*, 2205–2210.

Zimmerman, J. E., Knaus, W. A., Sharpe, S. M., Anderson, A. S., Draper, E. A., & Wagner, D. P. (1986). The use and implications of do-not-resuscitate orders in intensive care units. *Journal of the American Medical Association, 255*, 351–356.

10

HIV Testing: Patients' Rights versus Nurses' Rights

Ann Seidl

The epidemic of AIDS, or Acquired Immunodeficiency Syndrome, has resulted in major ethical and legal dilemmas for health care providers. There are also major economic considerations for clients, families, communities, health and social service delivery systems, and local, state, and federal governments both nationally and internationally. The development of policies regarding who should be tested for the HIV virus demands both a research base and the resolution of the complex ethical, legal, and economic issues.

KNOWLEDGE OF THE HIV VIRUS

AIDS is caused by a virus that attacks and destroys the immune system leaving the body vulnerable to diseases that it can normally repel. It is now common knowledge that AIDS is transmitted through semen and blood and through intimate sexual contact. It is also transmitted by sharing hypodermic needles and syringes, through blood transfusions, and transuterinely (see Table 10.1). Because of their exposure to body fluids, health care workers have had fears of being exposed to AIDS. Some have supported mandatory testing of patients, with the right of the health worker to know the results. On the other hand, as exemplified in the tragic case of Kimberly Bergalis, who was purported to have been infected by her dentist, David Acer, during routine dental care, patients and the general public have demanded mandatory testing of health care workers with disclosure.

TABLE 10.1 Body Fluids and Tissue From Which HIV Has Been Isolated or Transmission Documented

Body Fluid or Tissue	Virus Isolated	Transmission Documented	Occupation Transmission Documented
Blood	X	X	X
Serum	X		
Vaginal Secretions	X	X	
Semen	X	X	
Breast Milk	X	X	
In Utero		X	
Pleural Fluid		X	X
Alveolar Fluid	X		
Saliva	X		
Tears	X		
Urine	X		
Cerebrospinal Fluid	X		
Synovial Fluid	X		
Amniotic Fluid	X		
Brain	X		
Marrow	X		
Transplanted Kidney		X	
Transplanted Bone		X	
Transplanted Liver		X	

From Kelen, C. (1990). Human immunodeficiency virus and the emergency department: Risks and risk protection for health care providers. *Annals of Emergency Medicine*, 19 (3), 243.

Since HIV is not spread by casual encounters and no effective intervention to prevent HIV infection or cure AIDS exists, little public health rationale can be found to justify universal screening either of health care workers or patients, whether compulsory or voluntary (Howard, 1988).

Mandatory testing of health care workers is also highly debatable. Authorities supporting voluntary testing while opposing mandatory testing are the American Nurses Association, The Committee on National Strategy for AIDS, former Surgeon General Koop, the American Civil Liberties Union, the Centers for Disease Control, the American Medical Association, and Governor Cuomo, the Governor of New York State, the state with the largest number of AIDS cases and deaths. However, a warning is necessary. The *American Journal of Nursing* (Majority of RNs, 1991) stated that 93% of 1520 RNs surveyed would wear gloves while performing venipuncture on HIV-positive patients. However, only 59% would take that precaution if the patient's status was unknown. Furthermore, almost two-thirds of RNs surveyed thought that AIDS and hepatitis B are "equally transmissible." One in 20 RNs had been "stuck by a needle used on a patient whom they knew or suspected was HIV-positive," but under 20% correctly guessed the risk (under 1%) of acquiring HIV from one stick from a needle used on an AIDS patient.

MANDATORY TESTING

The general public believes that mandatory testing would contain the spread of AIDS, since early treatment and support would be available. This point of view is also substantiated by Lovejoy's research (1991) suggesting that early treatment slows the progress from the HIV antibody presence to full-blown AIDS from 4% to 2% per year of therapy. Early treatment with AZT also has been reported to delay the onset of dementia and retard the resistance to AZT. Others supporting mandatory testing argue that the statistics provided from such testing would provide a basis for the allocation of federal and local resources for both prevention and treatment efforts. Those found to be infected could be educated on how to prevent transmission of the virus and plan for anticipated health problems.

In general, employers in health institutions have been supportive of mandatory testing. Employee testing would allow employers to protect the health of the employee, maximizing both the patient's and the employee's protection. Some have suggested that knowing the status of all patients could reduce the cost of instituting universal precautions for all.

Landesman (1991) supports several guidelines that should direct policy. First, he recommends absolute honesty with the public. Second, he argues that consensus in the development of public health policy is necessary from the public health leadership. Third, in the formulation of public health policy, Landesman suggests we must educate ourselves and the public about the derivative and secondary implications of the policies put forth. Fourth, he describes the concept that directs policy development as the "least-restrictive alternative." Fifth, Landesman recommends that the formulation of public policy take the fears of the public at face value. Finally, he argues that the debate is driven by a perception of risk that is inappropriate to the level of that risk.

A survey (Tintinger & Simkins, 1989) of a nonrandom sample of 341 persons was conducted to investigate the relationship for various groups between attitudes regarding mandatory AIDS testing; attitudes toward the disease; sexual orientation and behavior; and attitudes toward homosexuals. Homosexual and bisexual respondents were less supportive of mandatory testing for anyone than were heterosexual respondents.

Greater homophobia and attitudes in favor of legal sanctions against persons with AIDS were correlated for heterosexual respondents, with attitudes supporting mandatory testing for everyone and homosexuals in particular. However, concern about contracting AIDS was unrelated to heterosexual attitudes favoring mandatory testing.

The issue comes down to protecting the rights of a few individuals versus protecting the society from the gravest public health threat. The obligation of the nation is to defend the safety and health of society as a whole. When the costs and benefits of mandatory testing for all health workers are weighed, some argue that the economic and psychosocial costs outweigh the benefits.

Risk to Patients

Public health and government officials have claimed that the risk of transmission from a health care worker to a patients is extraordinarily low, but not zero (see Table 10.2). One researcher (Fox, 1991) has suggested that lightning claims more lives each year than does AIDS acquired from health care workers, and that the risk of being hit by a careless motorist while on the way to the dentist's office is significantly higher than the likelihood of contracting HIV after arriving. However, Fox also reported that since the AIDS epidemic began, 6,782 health care workers with AIDS have been reported to the CDC. Furthermore, epidemiologists have estimated that approximately 15 million patients have been cared for by a doctor or dentist carrying the AIDS virus, only 5 infected patients have been reported.

Testing Reliability

The reliability of any HIV testing is questionable. Serum samples are screened with ELISA (enzyme-linked immuno-absorbent assay); if positive, a Western blot is completed to confirm the diagnosis. Tintinger and Simkins (1989) have indicated that the ELISA and Western blot tests for AIDS are not always completely predictive in high seroprevalence populations, let alone populations with lower seroprevalence. For example, in a population with a rate of approximately .03%, these tests will identify 380 false positive and 100 false negatives for every 1200 true positive cases. The false positive cases may be caused by an inconsistent interpretation of the Western blot; the false negative results may be caused by laboratory error. A false negative may provide a false sense of security, since it may take from 6–12 weeks to develop AIDS antibodies from the time of exposure, thus the negative test result of today may be the positive result of tomorrow.

TABLE 10.2 Risks to Patients Seeking Medical Care

Type	Magnitude
Risk of contracting HIV infection from a seropositive surgeon during invasive procedure	1 in 42,000 to 1 in 420,000 persons undergoing invasive procedure
Risk of contracting fatal hepatitis B virus infection from an HBeAg-positive surgeon during invasive procedures	1 to 76,000 to 1 in 1.4 million persons undergoing invasive procedure
Risk of contracting HIV infection after transfusion of blood with screening results negative for HIV	1 in 60,000 per unit of transfused blood
Risk of mortality due to general anesthesia	1 in 10,000 persons undergoing general anesthesia

From Lo, B. & Skinbrook, R. (1992) Health care workers infected with the human immuno-deficiency virsus. *Journal of the American Medical Association*, 267(8), 1101.

Impact of Testing on the Individual

Although it would be hoped that a person testing positive for HIV would refrain from high-risk activities to prevent transmission, this can not be assumed. There is some evidence that those who carry AIDS will take appropriate precautions. However, it is known that some infected individuals react completely differently, are angry at being infected, and desire to spread it to others. Mandatory testing may also force some individuals in high-risk groups "underground" to avoid being tested.

Mandatory Testing Implementation and Individual Rights

Public health researchers have found that 57% of physicians and 63% of nurses favored mandatory testing (Fox, 1991). An even greater proportion supported across-the-board testing of obstetric and surgical patients.

ETHICAL FRAMEWORK

To reach a decision on mandatory versus voluntary HIV testing for patients and health care workers, it is useful to use an ethical framework.

Consider the screening outcomes as benefits or harms.

Consider the distribution of benefit/harm between those tested and those not tested; the impact of screening on civil liberties; and these factors as they relate to the ethical principles of autonomy, beneficence, and justice.

Carol Levine, Executive Director, Citizens Commission on AIDS for New York City and Northern New Jersey, and Ronald Bayer, Associate Professor of the School of Public Health, Columbia University (1989) conclude that ethical principles may conflict. The principles of beneficence and harm may outweigh the need to obtain consent in some situations, but they never outweigh the obligation to treat persons with respect for their intrinsic worth and dignity. Levine and Bayer consider both the risks and benefits, drawing on the ethical principles of autonomy, beneficence, and justice, and reach the following conclusions:

1. There are now clinical and ethical grounds for establishing voluntary anonymous or confidential screening procedures in settings where individuals who may have been infected with HIV are treated.

2. Testing of competent adults for clinical purposes should be based on explicit informed consent.

3. There is no justification for mandatory screening on the grounds of therapeutic benefit.

4. Mandatory named reporting of those with HIV infection is unnecessary for clinical purposes and may be counterproductive.

5. High quality laboratory services must be used.

6. HIV-infected individuals should be protected against discrimination.

7. Screening programs to identify asymptomatic individuals for clinical purposes which do not at the same time plan for appropriate follow-up services fail to meet the ethical standards of justice or beneficence (Levine & Bayer, 1989, pp. 1663–1666).

ETHICAL PRINCIPLES GUIDING DECISIONMAKING

These ethical principles are derived from secular, religious, and constitutional traditions and are commonly applied to medicine, research, and public health. They can be used to examine specific situations to determine the ethical position.

Beneficence

Beneficence requires that we act on behalf of the interest and welfare of others. The obligations of beneficence apply to actions affecting both individuals and the community. Potential risks must be weighed against potential benefits and those actions with the most favorable risk-to-benefit ratio adopted. The justification for public health authority derives from both beneficence and the harm principle. Beneficence is the duty of the health professional to treat individuals with kindness. It requires us to "do good" without creating medical, social or psychological risk. Health care professionals have traditionally acted on behalf of the public good to protect individuals from unintentional harm and to provide care to the sick and disabled without regard to who they are and whatever they have done to contact disease. Mandatory testing for HIV diminishes the historically valued physician-patient relationship, supports involuntary self-incrimination, and sets the stage for cowardly acts involving the deprivation of rights.

Nonmaleficence

Nonmaleficence is the duty of the health professional to not harm or place an individual at risk. Nonmaleficence permits limitations in the liberties of individuals when their actions may harm another. Nurses and physicians take oaths to protect the public safety. It can be concluded that AIDS can be managed without mandatory testing because ethical behavior is based on knowledge of the facts and experience. It is the public's lack of knowledge and insistence of protection through legislation that justifies the development of alternatives to mandatory testing.

Autonomy

Autonomy is the right of an individual to self-determination and to be treated with respect. Infected health care workers do not merely lose their privacy leading to discrimination and stigmatization, but potentially lose their career and their livelihood. The disclosure of infection may evolve to a decision to limit the practice of the infected professional. This decision would significantly limit the pool of capable professionals. The loss of dedicated professionals through restrictive practice may also reduce the professionals available to care for infected patients. Gostin, Executive Director of the American Society of Law and Medicine states (1991) that employment discrimination is protected by federal legislation. Section 504 of the Federal Rehabilitation Act of 1973 and the Disabilities Act of 1990 support health care workers who have been denied or restricted in their practice. This is based on the assumption that individuals with AIDS have a handicap. The interpretation of the legislation is that the employment of an HIV-infected health care worker can only be limited if the worker exposes others to a "significant risk" and if such risk cannot be eliminated through reasonable accommodation. Furthermore, mandatory testing threatens health care workers and patients with involuntary termination of employment and meaningful involvement in the workplace, since career ladders of HIV seropositive workers have not been developed.

Justice

Justice requires that the benefits and burdens of particular actions be distributed fairly. Justice is also the basis for an individual's right to be treated fairly and without discrimination, and for the accessibility and allocation of resources equally distributed and without discrimination. Mandatory, serial testing of health care workers would appear to be a gross misuse of scarce resources when we consider the number of uninsured/underinsured people in this country.

Confidentiality

Mandatory AIDS testing raises major issues for those infected with the potential breach of confidentiality. Although there is great mental anguish and depression associated with positive HIV diagnoses, personal stigmatization and discrimination are also of great concern. Victims may lose their support networks, ability to work, medical insurance, income, savings, and housing.

Policies are being developed with two basic extremes. One is based on prejudice and irrational fear and requires testing and restrictions on a wide range of health professionals. The other is based on civil libertarian concerns and sets no limits. A solution based on how patients can best be protected against real risks without overreaction may be to set a professional rule with the following components (Gostin, 1991):

- Health care professionals should report their HIV-positive serologic status both to their employer and to their personal physician. Such information would become strictly confidential.
- HIV-infected professionals should be carefully monitored in the performance of their functions. This would include monitoring potentially impaired competence (e.g., fatigue and HIV dementia), infectious conditions (e.g., open sores on the skin and active tuberculosis), and compliance with rigorous infection control, including double gloving. Health care facilities might also be required to provide annual training in infection control. An HIV-infected professional could be asked to refrain from practicing noninvasive procedures only on individualized determinations of significant risk to patients.
- HIV-infected professionals should refrain from engaging in seriously invasive procedures.
- Health care facilities should develop policies and resources for retraining, support, counseling and compensation. (p. 665)

Gostin (1991) concludes: "The Public Health Service needs to draw a rational line before an irrational line is imposed by the courts and/or public opinion. The intimate nature of seriously invasive medical or dental procedures and the documentation of professional-to-patient transmission requires the adoption of this rational stand to maintain public confidence and patient safety" (p. 665).

LEGAL ARGUMENTS: MANDATORY HIV TESTING

Although ethical principle guides these decisions, legal issues must also be resolved.

Pro: Right to Know

It can be argued that health care workers and HIV-infected patients should be aware of their status and take extreme care to avoid transmitting the infection to their sexual contacts and to their patients.

Con: Civil Liberties

Implementation of mandatory testing may violate individual rights. It can be argued that a person has a constitutional right to privacy. This is in conflict with a government's obligation and power to protect the health and safety of its citizens. Individuals also have human and legal rights to body integrity, and this can justify the right to refuse testing. Furthermore, mandatory blood testing could qualify as search and seizure (Field, 1990). The Fourth Amendment to the Constitution requires compliance with a standard of reasonableness. These standards require the balance of the intrusion upon the individual's interests against the significance of the government's interests to justify such an intrusion. It can be argued that the risk that clients will contact AIDS is extremely low, and that the risk of disease transmission does not sufficiently justify a policy mandating blood testing.

Increased Liability

A Gallup poll found that 87% of laypeople surveyed believed that all doctors and nurses should be tested for AIDS. In Washington, a bill sponsored by Senator Jesse Helms would impose a 10-year sentence and a $10,000 fine on HIV-infected doctors who continue to practice without informing their patients. This bill passed the Senate by an overwhelming majority, 81–18, but is unlikely to become law (Greenberg, 1991, Hudson, 1991; p. 683). Employers can be found liable under common-law tort doctrines, under specific state statutes and municipal ordinances which prohibit the use of HIV antibody results in employment decisions, and under federal laws which prohibit discrimination on the basis of handicap. Tort actions for defamation, invasion of privacy, and negligent (or intentional) infliction of emotional distress can arise from wrongful disclosure of HIV screening results collected by employers and contained in employee records (Howard, 1988).

ECONOMIC ARGUMENTS

While there are ethical and legal components of decision making, there are also economic considerations.

Pro: Early Treatment

Supporters of mandatory testing suggest that there is a potential benefit in early treatment. Some studies suggest that early treatment slows the progress of HIV to AIDS. It also retards the resistance to AZT and delays the onset of dementia (Lovejoy, 1991), hypothetically allowing more years of independent self-care. This, of course, must be weighed against the myopathies that develop after 4 years of therapy and the lack of data suggesting that early treatment reduces mortality rates.

Enhanced Precautions

Strict adherence to infection control procedures and universal precautions is a major step toward AIDS control. The major element of universal precautions is the assumption that every patient is HIV-positive. The Centers for Disease Control's recommendations include the appropriate use of handwashing, protective barriers, and care in the use and disposal of needles and other sharp instruments. Health care workers who have lesions or weeping dermatitis should refrain from all direct patient care. Furthermore, these workers should not handle patient care equipment and devices used in performing invasive procedures until the condition resolves. Health care workers should also comply with current guidelines for disinfection and sterilization of reusable devices used in invasive procedures. It might be argued that treating every patient as if he or she is HIV-positive is more expensive than testing everyone so that you only have to use precautions, in terms of supplies, with those who actually are HIV positive. It may, then be cheaper to test everyone.

ELISA Test: Low Cost

The ELISA test costs about $3.00 with an additional $50.00 for the confirmatory Western blot. It is difficult, however, to make a convincing argument that there are economic benefits to mandatory testing. Testing to screen out infected blood from blood banks is clearly beneficial. Testing for research purposes allows the estimation of the incidence of HIV infection in certain subpopulations.

Con: Human/Social Cost

The diversion of significant sums away from HIV research, education, and medical care to operate a system of universal screening is socially wasteful.

Testing Not Absolute

Current screening programs for HIV infection use a sequence of screening tests, the enzyme-linked immunosorbent assay (ELISA) and the Western blot. Initially, serum samples are screened with the ELISA. The assay determines whether or not antibodies against HIV antigens are present. If the ELISA is positive, the sample is retested in duplicate using the same assay. If either of the retested samples is positive, the serum sample is tested by WESTERN blotting. This assay reveals the antibody profile of the sample. If the sample is reactive on Western blotting and is diagnostic of antibodies produced against key HIV antigens, the applicant is advised to submit a second new sample, which is also tested by Western blotting. Results of the Western blot test are crucial to diagnosis. However, the interpretation of these tests is inconsistent. The ELISA and Western blot tests have very low false positive rates, .005% to .0007% in some experienced laboratories. However, a false positive rate of .005% means that five of 100,000 people tested for HIV will be diagnosed with an infection, yet will not have it; 10 will be diagnosed who have the disease. It is known that there is an increase in the false positive rates with alcoholic disease, parenteral drug use, hemodialysis, multiple pregnancies, and multiple blood transfusions. The predictive value of a positive test result also depends on the prevalence of HIV infection in the population being tested (Lovejoy, 1991).

Cost Not Justified

The cost of mandatory testing is very high. The costs of testing programs must include not only the activities associated with testing itself, but also those activities associated with the results. Testing costs include enforcement of rules, laboratory fees, pretest and posttest counseling, and regulating laboratory standards. Activities related to testing results include segregation, detention, increased medical supervision, education, and prevention efforts. Data reported by Temple University (Eisenstaedt &

Getzen, 1988; Lovejoy, 1991) suggest that screening 10,000,000 individuals for HIV will cost $33,759,000. This assumes a fee schedule of $3.00 for the Elisa and $50.00 for the confirmatory Western blot. The cost of testing can be illustrated by the military expenditure of almost $20 million to perform HIV testing for 1 year alone (Santopoalo, 1989). If broad-based screening of the general population is considered, Field (1988) reported that of the 159,000 marriage license applicants in Illinois, 23 were found to be HIV-positive. The estimated cost for testing was $5.6 million which translates to $243,000 for each positive result. This expense for testing may be passed on to the public in the form of higher taxes and increased costs of health care. It is arguable that with limited resources, there is not enough money to fight this epidemic, money for preventative education, care for those that are infected, or research for cures.

THE PROFESSIONAL ORGANIZATION'S OPINION

The American Nurses Association (ANA) House of Delegates reaffirmed its opposition to mandatory testing and disclosure of human immunodeficiency virus (HIV) status of nurses and other health workers on June 28, 1991 at the ANA House of Delegates Meeting in Kansas City. They continue to support voluntary, anonymous testing and voluntary disclosure of the nurse's HIV status. The ANA Code for nurses indicates that the nurse "safeguards the client's right to privacy by ... protecting information of a confidential nature" (Palmer, 1991, p. 442). The Code also states that the nurse, as a client advocate, must protect the client "when health care and safety are affected by the ... practice of any person" (Palmer, 1991, p. 542). If a patient becomes exposed to a nurse's blood and/or body fluid in the course of receiving care, that nurse is ethically obligated to undergo testing for bloodborne pathogens, according to the ANA. The Association called for the development of a national consumer advisory statement outlining strict infection control procedures that should be used by all health care personnel. It further recommended that this consumer advisory statement be displayed in all health care settings and reviewed with patients. The ANA delegates agreed that patients have a right to be protected against transmission of HIV from their health care workers and that health care workers have a right to preserve their civil and human rights (Palmer, 1991). In passing the recommendations, the ANA delegates called for:

1. Continued development and implementation of national standards governing infection control techniques for invasive procedures wherever they are performed.

2. Extension of federal Occupational Health and Safety Administration standards requiring annual education on universal precautions and infection control for all health care workers.

3. An end to discrimination on the part of insurance companies toward people who test positive for HIV.

4. Support systems (administered by the state nurses associations) for HIV-positive nurses who confront personal and professional tragedies.

5. Presumptive compensability legislation for all nurses who, through occupational exposure, contract bloodborne pathogens.

6. Continued education for the public concerning the fact that HIV and AIDS transmission occurs primarily through unsafe sexual activity and IV drug use with shared needles (Palmer, 1991, p. 541).

THE CENTERS FOR DISEASE CONTROL

The CDC does not advocate mandatory testing of the health care workers because

> The current assessment of the risk that infected health care workers will transmit HIV or HBV (Hepatitis B virus) to patients during exposure-prone procedures does not support the diversion of resources that would be required to implement mandatory testing programs. (Reeder, 1991, p. 692).

(See Table 10.3).

The infection rate has remained constant at approximately 0.40%, or 1 infection for every 250 percutaneous exposures (Beekman, Fahey, Gerberding, & Henderson, 1990).

(See Table 10.4).

LEGAL IMPLICATIONS FOR HEALTH CARE WORKERS

The following questions are frequently asked by health care workers concerned with HIV infections. There are some suggested answers.

Can you sue the hospital if you HIV sero-convert during employment? Proof of causation is the difficulty in suing in this area. Health care professionals must prove that their sero-positivity was caused directly by a needlestick or puncture with a device used on an HIV-infected patient. This may prove difficult. If a hospital provides workers' compensation for occupational illness, employees are precluded by law from suing the hospital in a tortious action (Morthorst, 1991).

TABLE 10.3 Summary of Published Prospective Studies of the Risk for Occupational/Nosocomial Transmission of HIV-1 Following Percutaneous Exposure

Number of studies	14
Number of participants	1,962
Number of percutaneous exposures	2,008
Number of seroconversions	6
Infection rate per participant	0.32%
Infection rate per exposure	0.31%

From Beekman, S., Fahey, B., Gerberding, J., & Henderson, D. (1990). "Risky business: Using necessarily imprecise casualty counts to estimate occupational risks for HIV-1 infection." *Infection Control and Hospital Epidemiology, 11*(7), 371–378.

Can you get fired for refusing HIV testing or for being HIV-positive? The impact of the CDC guidelines released in July 1991 regarding HIV screening of health care professionals was not clear at the time of this writing. However, in Lecket v. Board of Commissioners of Hospital District No. 1, 1989 the court upheld a ruling that the firing of an LPN for failure to comply with the hospital's request for HIV antibody testing did not violate the nurse's civil rights. The nurse, a known homosexual, lived with a roommate who had died from AIDS. On the advice of hospital counsel, the executive director of the hospital asked the nurse to submit to an AIDS test. The nurse informed the hospital that he had been tested elsewhere for HIV but he refused to reveal the results. The court rejected the plaintiff's argument that he was discriminated against as a handicapped person. The court reasoned that he was fired for failing to submit the test results and not on the basis of the results themselves. The court also

TABLE 10.4 Gender of Health Care Workers (HCWs) Reported with Possible Occupational HIV-1 Infection Compared with All U.S. Health Care Workers

Category	N [in millions]	Men	Women
All U.S. HCWs	5.7	23%	77%
Documented seroconversions	27	11%	89%
Reported prevalent positives	9	44%	56%
Other anecdotal reports	26	58%	42%
AIDS in HCWs with no identified risk	66	71%	29%

From Beekman, S., Fahey, B., Gerberding, J., & Henderson, D. (1990). "Risky business: Using necessarily imprecise casualty counts to estimate occupational risks for HIV-1 infection." *Infection Control and Hospital Epidemiology, 11*(7), 377.

concluded that the right to know the plaintiff's health status, especially in light of his association with an AIDS patient, outweighed his right to privacy (Morthorst, 1991).

Can you be sued and found liable for transmitting HIV infection to a patient? Although there is no case history on this aspect, the answer is YES (Morthorst, 1991). If the patient can prove that he or she is not in any high-risk group for contracting AIDS and can trace a causal link back to the health care professional, then the patient may be able to win a lawsuit. The pursuit of these cases is under civil law and is still untested regarding health care workers. Twenty states have enacted statutes that permit prosecution of persons whose behaviors pose risk of HIV transmission. If a health care worker knows that he or she is HIV-positive and knowingly participates in invasive procedures on patients, then he or she possibly could be charged with a criminal act.

There are cases starting to appear in the judicial system surrounding these issues. In one case, Halverson v. Brand, Ms. Halverson, a nurse, sued a patient's physician for not informing her of their patient's diagnosis of AIDS (1986). She alleged negligence on the part of the physician and "emotional trauma" for not informing her of this diagnosis until after she had participated in an invasive diagnostic procedure on the patient without the use of protective gloves when a cut was on her hand. The trial court dismissed the petition and the dismissal was upheld at the appellate level. It remains for the Pennsylvania Supreme Court to decide if Halverson has a right to proceed with her case. Although she was clearly in the wrong for not wearing gloves and other protective gear during the procedure, if the facts are accurate, the response to Halverson's suit is thought-provoking.

AIDS, the clinical end point of the continuum of HIV infection, is a reportable disease in all 50 states and U.S. territories. Standardized reports of people who meet a uniform AIDS case definition are sent without names from state, local, and territorial health departments to CDC, which has maintained a national surveillance system since 1981. Health care workers with AIDS are similar in age and gender to non health care workers but are more likely to be white. About 70% of the health care workers with AIDS have died. In comparison to other AIDS patients, health care workers are more likely to be homosexual/bisexual men (70% vs. 60%) and less likely to be intravenous drug users (7% vs. 22%) (Ciesielski, Gooch, Hammett, & Metler, 1991) (See Table 10.5).

In the last several years, Arkansas and Missouri have required patients to tell health care workers their HIV status before an invasive procedure. Oregon, West Virginia, and Virginia have given patients the right to learn the HIV status of a health care worker following a significant exposure. Twenty-eight states give health care workers the right to learn a patient's

TABLE 10.5 Adult AIDS Cases Reported to CDC Through March, 31, 1991

Transmission mode	NOT HCW*[a] (percentage)	HCW[b] (percentage)
Homosexual/Bisexual male	60	70
Heterosexual IV drug user	22	7
Homosexual/Bisexual IV drug user	7	7
Hemophiliac	1	1
Heterosexual contact	5	7
Transfusion recipient	2	2
Other	<1	<1
Undetermined	3	6

*HCW = Health Care Worker
[a]n = 129,181
[b]n = 6,265
From "Dentists, allied professionals with AIDs" by C. Ciesielski, B. Gooch, T. Hammett, and R. Mether, 1991, *Journal of the American Dental Association, 122*, p. 44.

TABLE 10.6 Recommendations for Health Care Facilities Where Invasive Procedures are Performed

Should provide

- Annual training for all personnel engaged in invasive procedures in barrier techniques, universal blood and body fluid precautions, and other scientifically accepted infection control practices.
- Information on HIV risk factors and the merits of voluntary, confidential or anonymous counseling and testing as a personal health measure.
- Information on the availability of voluntary, confidential or anonymous HIV counseling and testing for staff.
- Policy guidelines for the prevention of transmission of blood borne pathogens, including HIV, during invasive procedures, and guidelines for improving infection control practices, where indicated. Also, facilities have an obligation to provide effective barrier protection equipment and supplies.
- Procedures for the evaluation of work limitations for HIV-infected workers showing evidence of functional impairment or of inability to adhere to standard infection control practices.
- An employee health designee (EHD) responsible for the monitoring of all health workers whose compromised function or health condition possesses significant risk to patients at the facility.

New York State Department of Health Policy Statements and Guidelines Health Care Facilities & HIV-Infected Medical Personnel. By New York State Department of Health Memorandum, p. 3.

HIV status following a significant exposure. Professional societies will have to develop a specific list of exposure-prone procedures, such as obstetric or cardiac surgery. New York State has developed recommendations for health care facilities (see Table 10.6), and provided guidelines for modification or reassignment of duties for all health care workers, including health care workers with HIV (see Tables 10.7 and 10.8).

The complex legal, ethical, and economic issues surrounding decisions regarding testing of health care workers and patients as well as the general public are continually evolving. Summaries of the major pros and cons for addressing HIV-infected health care workers by adding to universal precautions, by voluntary testing and voluntary abstention from invasive procedures, by mandatory testing and mandatory abstention from invasive procedures are seen in Table 10.9.

TABLE 10.7 New York State Recommendations

HIV-infected professionals should continue all professional practice for which they are qualified, with rigorous adherence to universal precautions and scientifically accepted infection control practices. Decisions about work responsibilities of HIV-infected individuals with evidence of functional impairment or lack of infection control competence should continue to be made on a case-by-case basis, involving the worker's personal physician.

From AIDS: Debate on infection control guidelines shifts to Congress by T. Hudson, 1991. *Hospitals*, *65*, 32. Reprinted from *Hospitals*, Vol. 65, No. 17, by permission, September 5, 1991, copyright 1991, American Hospital Publishing, Inc.

TABLE 10.8 Factors Considered on the Potential Limitation, Modification or Reassignment of Duties for all Health Care Workers, Including Health Care Workers with HIV Infection, Include the Following:

- Illness that may interfere significantly with the health care worker's ability to provide quality care. Both physical and mental competence are to be considered.
- The immunologic status of the health care worker and susceptibility to infectious diseases.
- The presence of exudative or weeping lesions.
- Functional inability to perform assigned tasks or regular duties.
- Documentation of evidence of previous transmission of blood borne pathogens, including HBV.
- Noncompliance with established guidelines to prevent transmission of the disease.

New York State Department of Health Policy Statements and Guidelines Health Care Facilities & HIV-Infected Medical Personnel. By New York State Department of Health Memorandum (Januray 1991) p. 3.

TABLE 10.9 Summary of the Major Pros and Cons of Alternative Options for Addressing HIV-Infected Health Care Workers

Option 1. Adherence to the universal precautions

Pros	Cons
• Consistent with evidence on the minimal risks of transmission and demonstrated effectiveness of universal precautions at reducing the risk of transmission.	• Poses potential hospital liability for suits from patients for harm or emotional distress.
• Consistent with the methods used for preventing the transmission of other blood-borne diseases in hospitals.	• May generate bad publicity given public belief that the fatality of AIDS necessitates more drastic measures for preventing transmission.
• Protects health care workers from invasion of privacy, discrimination, and the loss of their livelihood.	• May not offer adequate protection to patients in light of the uncertainty about the risks and methods of HIV transmission, particularly when invasive procedures are performed.
• Decreases risk of hospital liability for employment discrimination, breaches of confidentiality, and other intrusions on doctors' right to privacy.	• Denies patients a right to know the HIV status of their doctors and make an informed decision about allowing the doctor to perform invasive procedures.
• Avoids the substantial social and economic costs of greater restrictions on the rights of HIV-infected HCWs to practice.	

Option 2. Voluntary testing/voluntary abstention from invasive procedures or informed consent

Pros	Cons
• Protects and respects patients' rights to know and to give informed consent.	• Risks infringing on the rights of doctors.
• Reduces possibility of patient liability lawsuits.	• May be unnecessary, unjustified by the evidence to date and inconsistent with the controls used to prevent transmission of other infectious diseases.
• Focuses on adding safeguards to invasive procedures which do pose the greatest risk of transmission to patient.	• Poses potential liability for employment discrimination against HIV-infected health care workers.
• Avoids the greater intrusions on privacy and practical difficulties associated with mandatory testing programs.	• Imposes substantial social and economic costs.
• Likely to be good for public relations.	• Less effective at identifying infected practitioners than mandatory testing programs.

Option 3. Mandatory Testing/Mandatory Abstention from Invasive Procedures

Pros	Cons
• Provides strongest guarantee of patients' rights not to be operated on by HIV-infected health care workers. • More effective at identifying and restricting infected practitioners than voluntary testing. • Likely to be good for public relations unless the severity generates a backlash from the medical community. • Reduces the possibility of patient liability lawsuits.	• Poses the most substantial intrusion on the privacy of infected health care workers of the policies being advocated. • May be unnecessary, unjustified by the evidence to date and inconsistent with the controls used to prevent transmission of other infectious diseases. • Poses potential liability for employment discrimination against HIV infected health care workers. • Raises practical difficulties of determining whom to test, how often to test, and who should pay for testing. • Costly and not clearly outweighed by the benefits given the minimal risks of transmission. • Imposes substantial social and economic costs.

From Options for addressing HIV-infected health care workers and analysis of the legal and policy implications by W. H. E. Von Oehsen & S. E. Hendrickson (June 24, 1991). Memorandum pp. 15–17.

TOPICS FOR DISCUSSION

1. Should all health care workers be required to be tested for the HIV virus?
2. Would you be legally liable if you were HIV-positive and infected a patient? Explain.
3. How likely is infection of a patient by a health care worker?
4. Review and define the following ethical principles; beneficence, nonmaleficence, autonomy, and justice. How do they relate to the issue of mandatory HIV testing for health care workers?
5. How accurate are the current tests for HIV?

REFERENCES

Beekman, S., Fahey, B., Gerberding, J., & Henderson, D. (1990). Risky business: Using necessarily imprecise casualty counts to estimate occupational risks for HIV-1 infection. *Infection Control & Hospital Epidemiology, 11*, 371–378.

Ciesielski, C., Gooch, B., Hammett, T., & Metler, R. (1991). Dentists, allied profes-
   sionals with AIDS. *Journal of the American Dental Association, 122,* 42–44.
Eisenstaedt, R., & Getizen, T. (1988). Screening Blood Donors for Human Immu-
   nodeficiency Antibody: Cost Benefit Analysis. *American Journal of Public
   Health, 78,* 450–454.
Field, M. (1990). Testing for AIDS: Uses and abuses. *American Journal of Law and
   Medicine, 16,* 34–106.
Fox, C. H. (1991). AIDS transmission: Hazardous health care? *Harvard Health Let-
   ter, 17,* 4–6.
Gostin, L. (1991). The HIV-infected health care professional: Public policy, dis-
   crimination, and patient safety. *Archives of Internal Medicine, 151,* 663–665.
Greenberg, D. (1991). Racheting up the AIDS hysteria. *The Lancet, 338,* 683–684.
Halverson v. Brand, 362 PA Super Ct 628, 520 A 2d 67 (1986), No. 121 (PA Supreme
   Court, April 1988).
Halverson v. Brand as cited in Brent, N. (1990). Confidentiality and HIV status:
   The nurse's right to know. *Home Health Care Nurse, 8,* 6–8.
Howard, J. (1988). HIV screening: Scientific, ethical, and legal issues. *The Journal
   of Legal Medicine, 9,* 601–610.
Hudson, T. (1991). AIDS: Debate on infection control guidelines shifts to Congress.
   Hospitals, 65, 30–33.
Kelen, G. (1990). Human immunodeficiency virus and the emergency department:
   Risks and risk protection for health care providers. *Annals of Emergency
   Medicine, 19*(3), 242–248.
Landesman, S. (1991). The HIV-positive health professional: Policy options for
   individuals, institutions, and states. *Archives of Internal Medicine, 151,* 655–
   657.
Lecket v. Board of Commissioners of Hospital District No 1, 909 F 2d 820 (5th Cir
   1990).
Levine, C., & Bayer, R. (1989). The ethics of screening for early intervention in
   HIV disease. *American Journal of Public Health, 79,* 1661–1667.
Lo, B., & Skinbrook, R. (1992). Health Care Workers Infected with Human immu-
   nodeficiency virus. Journal of the American Medical Association 267, 1100–
   1105.
Lovejoy, N. (1991). Arguments against mandatory screening for HIV in low-preva-
   lence areas. *Journal of the Association of Nurses in AIDS Care, 2,* 7–15.
Majority of RNs favor mandatory testing for AIDS. (1991, August). *American Jour-
   nal of Nursing,* 11.
Morthorst, M. (1991). AIDS, HIV infection and health care professionals. *Ameri-
   can Operating Room Nurses Journal, 54,* 597–601.
New York State Department of Health Policy, *Statement and Guidelines: Health
   Care Facilities and HIV infected Medical Personnel* Spring, 1991, p. 1–4
Palmer, P. (1991). American Nurses Association delegates issue HIV recommen-
   dations, finalize affiliate status fee structure. *American Operating Room
   Nurses Journal, 54,* 541–545.
Santopoalo, T. (1989). Mandatory testing for AIDS antibody. *Journal of Commu-
   nity Health Nursing, 6*(4), 231–244.
Tintinger, J., & Simkins, L. (1989). Mandatory AIDS testing: Factors influencing
   public opinions. *Psychological Reports, 65,* 835–843.
Von Oehsen, W. H. E., & Hendrickson, S. E. (1991, June 24). *Memorandum options
   for addressing HIV infected healthcare workers and analysis of the legal and
   policy implications.* Memorandum. Washington, DC: National Association of
   Public Hospitals.

11

Institutionalization versus Noninstitutionalization of the Elderly: A Major Issue in Nursing

Linda M. Janelli

There are many critical issues facing a graying American Society, but none seems to have as much impact as the issue of institutionalization, which affects not only the elderly individual, but the whole family structure. Even though the elderly population is rapidly increasing, currently, only a small percentage live in institutional settings. However, this trend is predicted to be changing. Almost half of all Americans who turned 65 in 1990 will spend some time in a nursing home before they die. The estimate is that 1 in 7 men and 1 in 3 women will face institutionalization. By the year 2040 there will be approximately 5.2 million elderly in nursing homes. Not only will more older persons be residing in institutions, but more of them will be displaying a greater level of disability (Murtaugh, Kemper & Spillman, 1990).

As the elderly population continues to burgeon the demand for community resources and nursing home care will become even more pronounced. The concern for quality care in institutions needs to be addressed. Some nursing home philosophies have attempted to put less emphasis on a custodial care model, and more emphasis on a rehabilitative model, which stresses individual needs, flexibility, and family involvement. There are interrelationships between an aging society and the health care that such a society can provide. These interrelationships can affect public policy and moral and ethical considerations, as well as families acting as caregivers (Selker & Broski, 1988).

This chapter will focus on describing institutional settings, those who reside there, what factors lead to institutionalization, how the elderly adapt to nursing homes, alternatives to institutionalization, and finally nursing's role in this complex issue.

THE DEMOGRAPHIC IMPERATIVE

Projections for the population demonstrate that the number of elderly will continue to increase. In 1900, the median age at death was 58. The median age at death is now over 79, and by the year 2000 will be approximately 82. This will mean a gain of longevity roughly equal to that which occurred from the time of Christ up to the year 1900 (Ansello, 1991). By the year 2050, those 65 years of age and older will account for 25% of the population (Selker & Broski, 1988).

An even more enormous growth is expected between 1990 and 2010 in the number of persons aged 85 and older. This old-old group is anticipated to increase, as seen in Table 11.1, by 50% or more in 13 states (Kovar & Feinleib, 1991). Demographics also reveal that this older population will be increasingly female. Many women living at the beginning of the twentieth century never lived to experience menopause; today they reach the age of 75 or 85—some eight years longer than most men (Porcino, 1983). Not only are there more elderly women, but almost 40% of them live alone. There is also a higher rate of arthritis, osteoporosis, hip fracture, and hypertensive disease among older women (U.S. Senate Special Committee on Aging, 1984).

Chronic conditions such as arthritis, heart conditions, and visual and hearing conditions are more prominent among the elderly. Forty percent

Table 11.1 Projected Population Increases From 1990 to 2010 Among Those 85 and Older

State	Projected increase
Alaska	100%
Arizona	80%
Delaware	50%
Florida	75%
Georgia	60%
Hawaii	80%
Maryland	50%
Nevada	86%
New Mexico	53%
North Carolina	61%
South Carolina	67%
Utah	57%
Virginia	52%

Source M. Kovar and M. Fernleib (1991). Older Americans present a double challenge: Preventing disability and providing care. *American Journal of Public Health, 81,* 287–288.

of those 65 to 84 years of age and 60% of those 85 and over experience limitation in their activities of daily living due to a chronic illness. Because of these chronic conditions, the elderly are more likely to use health services. Many of them, however, are either underinsured or uninsured against catastrophic and long-term care costs (Selker & Broski, 1988).

DEFINING INSTITUTIONALIZATION

The terms "institutionalization" and "long-term care" are often used synonymously. Nursing home institutions have been described as "human junkyards," "warehouses," "dehumanizing," and "depersonalizing." An institution can be defined as a social unit devoted primarily to the achievement of specific goals. There are three goals generally associated with long-term care: 1) to delay the onset of preventable disease in healthy adults, 2) to lengthen the period of functional independence in the elderly with chronic disease, and 3) to improve quality of life (Kart, Metress & Metress, 1988).

Erving Goffman (1961) defined a "total" institution as a place where persons are segregated from society, treated alike, and required to do the same thing together at a prearranged time. Goffman drew attention to the effect that institutions such as nursing homes could have on individuals, especially when they are excluded from the decisions made regarding their fate. Goffman believes that institutions strip away an individual's self-identity in order to better manage them. Stripping includes loss of personal possessions, clothing, and loss of privacy.

Not all nursing homes or long-term care facilities are total institutions as described by Goffman. They often differ in the quality and type of care they provide. The nursing home institutions may provide custodial care, medical care, or a combination of both. They may be proprietary homes operated under private commercial licenses, nonprofit homes operated under voluntary auspices, or government homes run by local, state, or federal agencies. They also vary in the number of beds and the types of persons who reside there.

Most nursing homes are for profit (proprietary). About one-third of all nursing homes are located in the north central region of the country which geographically also contains a larger percentage of older residents. Nursing homes can also be classified by their certification status. There are skilled nursing facilities (SNF) and intermediate care facilities (ICF). Those classified as SNFs provide a full range of medical and nursing services, whereas those classified as ICFs provide for custodial care, such as assistance with personal hygiene and administration of medication (Kart et al., 1988). A nationwide survey by the Agency for Health Care

Policy Research in Rockville, Maryland, questions whether nursing homes, which currently charge approximately $25,000 a year per person, should remain the main mechanism of care for the elderly. Medicaid, the principal method of public financing of nursing homes, in 1988 paid for more than 44% of all nursing home expenses (Lamb, 1992).

ENTERING AN INSTITUTION

In 1985, the nursing home population was 1.3 million or 5% of the elderly. By the year 2000 2 million will be living in nursing homes, with 4.4 million by 2040 (Zarle, 1989). Almost 81% of those admitted to a nursing home are admitted for physical reasons such as cerebral vascular accidents, heart disease, incontinence, arthritis, and dementia. The "typical" nursing home resident has been described as being white, widowed, and a woman.

There is low utilization of nursing homes by non whites. Non whites comprise only 8% of the institutional population. This low utilization may be due to cultural differences in attitudes toward institutionalization or informal caregiving. Another explanation is that non whites are being denied access due to discrimination by nursing home administrators against minorities or Medicaid patients, or inability of minorities to pay for care (Murtaugh et al., 1990).

A disproportionate number of those in nursing homes are women—more than 71%. This can be explained by the fact that in the older age group, women survive longer than men. Being a widow and living alone are both factors that place women at risk for institutionalization. Finally, more than 4 out of 5 residing in nursing homes are over the age of 75 (Kart et al., 1988).

One study has noted (Smallegan, 1985) that the decision to enter a nursing home is usually due to inadequacy of either finances, health, social supports, emotional strength, or any other ability to cope. Many of those admitted to a nursing home have complex physical and social problems. This study breaks the myth that families use nursing homes to "dump" their family members. It is only when families can no longer manage problems because they exceed their abilities, resources, or emotional strength that nursing home placement becomes necessary.

In fact, 80% of the services that the elderly receive in the community is the result of family support, not medical or nursing support. Families are not undergoing dissolution; rather, individuals are surviving longer with chronic disabilities. The literature and the media have popularized the myth of three- and four-generation families residing under one roof, however, this was not true in the past. The intergenerational family is becoming more of a reality today because younger families cannot afford their own homes and because of the financial burden of institutionalization.

Johnson and Werner (1982) found in their study that prior to institutionalization, family members reported an average of 4.2 problems for each person entering a nursing home. The most common symptoms seen in a family member prior to nursing home admission included: loss of control of urine, loss of ability to walk, disorientation to time and place, loss of memory, and severe physical illness. Although chronic illness is common to both community-based and institutionalized elderly, what distinguishes these two groups is the impact and disability that occurs as a result of the chronic condition. One fourth of the elderly residing in nursing homes are dependent in all six activities of daily living: feeding, dressing, bathing, continence, using the toilet, and mobility. Ninety-three percent of the elderly in nursing homes require assistance in at least one activity of daily living, compared with only 9% of the noninstitutionalized elderly (Brody & Foley, 1985). Even when the need for institutionalization becomes apparent to family members or to the elderly person themselves, the decision is not an easy one to make. Many families are ambivalent about nursing home placement because of feelings of guilt; they may view themselves as failing somehow, or may hold the same negative attitudes as general society towards institutions.

NURSING HOME ADJUSTMENT

Relocation into a nursing home is one of the major events in a person's life. A person entering a nursing home faces many stressful losses. There can be loss of friendships and familiar places, loss of personal possessions, and loss of control. The elderly person can no longer decide when to get up, when to eat, what to wear—choices and privacy become limited. Relationships with family members may also change and contribute to the elderly person's loss of self-esteem (Mikhail, 1992). Studies on the elderly who have resided in a variety of institutional settings seem to indicate that they are more likely to be maladjusted and depressed, have a lower range of interests and activity, and are more likely to die sooner than those elderly living in the community (Kant et al., 1988).

The elderly are in a better position to accept nursing home placement when they view it as legitimate or voluntary, desirable or important, and reversible. Successful adaptation can occur when the elderly person who is cognitively intact begins to realize that their health is failing, they can no longer manage their own activities of daily living, or that their spouse or caregiver's health is in jeopardy. An individual's involvement in the decisionmaking process can greatly enhance their adjustment to a nursing home. If however, the individual is not a part of the decisionmaking process he or she may feel abandoned, hurt, and angry. They may respond by withdrawing, by being demanding, or acting out against family or staff. The adaptation can also be affected by unrealistic expectations of the family or the elderly. Poorly controlled medical conditions may become stabilized during institutionalization, but the underlying physiologic condition is not going to change. Family members who have resolved their own feelings and conflicts about their parent's mortality can be instrumental in facilitating adjustment to the nursing home environment (Chenitz, 1983).

Brooke (1989) has identified four major phases in the process of adapting to a nursing home: disorganization, reorganization, relationship building, and stabilization.

Disorganization, sometimes referred to as translocation syndrome, is characterized by feelings of displacement, vulnerability, and abandonment. For most elderly residing in a nursing home this phase lasts only about 6 to 8 weeks. They may be anxious, apprehensive, or despondent, and may express death wishes. Fatigue, restlessness, and loss of appetite are frequent symptoms.

Reorganization refers to the phase in which the individual attempts to find meaning, and to legitimize his/her life in the nursing home. This phase usually occurs in the second or third month. During reorganization the elderly person is involved in problem solving, identifying preferred care and directing others in that care, and resolving or justifying their residence in a nursing home. Common signs seen during this phase are questioning about care, complaining about limited space, and explaining needs to new staff.

Relationship building begins generally around the third month and is characterized by the development of emotional ties with others who are institutionalized as well as with staff. During this phase individuals squabble with each other and identify favorite staff members. Grief is often felt when a fellow institutionalized elder dies.

Stabilization is the last phase when the elderly person has worked through some losses, established working relationships with staff, developed personal ties and has settled in. This phase generally occurs within 3 to 6 months. The individual begins to view the new environment as home. The challenge of the stabilization phase is for the elderly person to conform to the nursing home without losing their self-identity.

Almost all elderly, if given a choice, would prefer to remain in their own homes, maintaining a life-style as independent as possible. However, achieving this goal is not always practical. The following example concerns an elderly woman who with the assistance of her family struggled to maintain her status at home until well-coordinated care was no longer available.

CASE EXAMPLE

Mrs. M.A. is an 83-year-old white widow living in a large Victorian home with an unmarried daughter. Her diagnoses include left-sided cerebral vascular accident, cataracts bilaterally, prolapsed uterus, osteoarthritis, and a repaired right hip fracture.

Assessment Parameters for Institutionalization

1. *Environmental assessment.* Is alone during the day while daughter works. Bedrooms are located on second floor. Spends most of day in living room with a bathroom facility near by. Becoming increasingly difficult to use walker.

2. *Activities of daily living status.* Requires someone to prepare all meals, administer medication, dressing, and bathing. Needs assistance with transferring, ambulating, and toileting. Sometimes is incontinent and wears adult diapers. Can feed self but has a poor appetite.

3. *Mental status.* Has focal defects, including poor short-term memory, poor judgement, and limited reasoning ability. Does not like being in a room by herself and will call out her daughter's name. Can use the phone, but has called the police stating she was being held a prisoner. States a strong desire to stay in her own home even though she realizes the stress this creates for her daughter.

4. *Lifestyle assessment.* Drove a car until she was 78 years old. Helped her husband with running of a grocery store but has been primarily a housewife. Has two sisters and a brother in the same city. Recreational activities prior to present health problems included reading, watching television, and exploring new restaurants and shops.

5. *Social support status.* Has only a few friends who maintain contact by phone. When possible was going to church weekly with daughter. Had a Friendly Visitor twice per week for a few hours. Went to an adult day care 2 days a week when she was able to go by wheelchair. A home health agency provided an aide 3 days a week. Could no longer be left in the house alone. Sometimes a sitter would be obtained by the daughter from among church members to provide her with some respite on the weekend.

6. *Family status.* Daughter provides the most support. Changed jobs to be closer to home and works only half days Mondays, Wednesdays, and Fridays. Daughter did all food shopping and preparation as well as housekeeping. However, she does not drive. Has one son who is a lawyer with a family of his own. Devoted to his mother and visited every day and would call each evening.

7. *Recent life changes.* Lost her husband 2 years ago and shortly after had a stroke.

8. *Sensory impairment.* Hemiparesis (left-sided), only has weakness, not true paralysis. Hearing intact, but vision and depth perception are poor. Has glasses but states they do not help. Has difficulty expressing herself and naming objects.

Evaluation

Although the care at home for Mrs. M. A. was less expensive than institutionalization, the psychological stress of maintaining her at home was affecting her daughter, who was diagnosed with hypertension. Mrs. M.A. was experiencing numerous falls at home, especially since she would attempt to get up unassisted. She was reluctant to go to bed at night and would want to be dressed at 3 or 4 a.m. She experienced one fall that required sutures to her scalp and upon admission to the Emergency Room she was also diagnosed as having a trans-ischemic attack (TIA). Mrs. M.A. was hospitalized for further tests and with the physicians' and social worker's input the family decided the time was appropriate to begin the search for nursing home placement. After 6 months on an alternate level of care unit at a hospital she was relocated to a skilled nursing facility.

COMMUNITY-BASED CARE: AN ALTERNATIVE TO INSTITUTIONALIZATION

As previously stated, 95% of all elderly persons, if given the chance, would prefer to reside in their own homes. But in reality there is often a problem of matching the need of the elderly with accessible services. There are many barriers that can prevent the elderly from obtaining needed services such as Medicare, attitudes towards the elderly, and cultural and psychological barriers. Although Medicare has made available medical services to the elderly who would not receive these services otherwise, there are limitations. Only about 44% of the medical costs of the elderly is paid through Medicare. Medicare focuses more on acute rather than chronic care and will not, for example, pay for eye and hearing examinations, nor for orthopedic shoes and false teeth (Kart et al., 1988).

Geographic proximity to services can be a problem, especially for the elderly living in rural areas. Urban areas have been better able to provide a greater variety of services at a lower cost. Transportation also affects utilization of services. Lack of knowledge about the services are available in a community, as well as how to access those services can be frustrating and time-consuming (Dunkle, 1988). Studies have indicated that when elderly living in the community are asked what existing services there are available to them, the majority have no idea.

A significant amount of informal care is provided by family caregivers who are responsible for maintaining the elderly in their community setting. The estimate is that 1 in 4 workers has some responsibility for an elderly person, either providing daily care or regularly monitoring, shopping, or transporting. About 6 million elderly are receiving caregiving which allows them to remain in the community. The most common caregivers for the elderly are spouses, who themselves are aging, and adult children who are becoming old themselves and dealing with their own retirement and health issues. Research data indicates that in some families one individual is "elected" to the role of designated caregiver. Gender is often linked to the responsibilities designated to the caregiver, with daughters, wives, sisters, and other female family members assuming the hands-on-care and sons, husbands, brothers, and other men assuming responsibilities for financial management (Ansello, 1991; Phillips, 1989).

Formal community-based services that are available to the elderly vary according to geography, policies, and finances. These support services have been designed to provide an alternative to institutionalization as well as to aid the informal caregiving structure. The following formal services will be identified in order to demonstrate the range of services available: home health care, senior centers/nutrition centers, meals-on-wheels, adult day care, respite care, and hospice care. This is not meant to be an all-inclusive list.

Home Health Care

Home health care's goal is to provide coordinated multidisciplinary services which may include skilled nursing as well as social casework, mental health, legal, financial and personal care, and household management. Under most home health care programs, a registered nurse conducts an individualized assessment of each elderly person who requests home care, so that services and home health aides can be matched with the needs of the client (Crossman, 1991).

The total public health care funding for home care has been relatively small since most of the federal and states monies have been diverted to nursing home and acute care hospital settings. Approximately 80% of the elderly receiving home care are post-hospital referrals; the others are referred by a physician after an episode of illness or by family or friends who need help in providing care.

There are a variety of home health care agencies which include hospital-based, private profit and nonprofit agencies, and public agencies, such as public health and social service departments. Hospital-based home health agencies provide several advantages in that they can assure continuity of care from hospital to home. With patient stays in hospitals becoming shorter due to diagnostic related groups (DRGs), hospital-based home care has helped hospitals to control inpatient costs. Proprietary home care agencies or profit making agencies are licensed by individual states for governmental reimbursement. There has been increasing concern over the number of proprietary agencies, which have grown over 8 times that of hospital-based and nonprofit agencies. The major roles that nurses play in home health care include providing direct care, managing and supervising nonprofessionals, and coordinating services (Dunkle, 1988; Matteson & McConnell, 1988).

Senior Centers/Nutrition Centers

Senior centers provide an avenue for the elderly to socialize by providing a variety of recreational activities such as card playing, arts and crafts, singing, and dancing. These centers may function as a means to assist the elderly in gaining access to other community services. Some senior centers also provide educational activities to assist the elderly to better cope with chronic conditions. Health-related assessments may be conducted by nurses, physicians and other health professionals in such areas as hypertension, oral cancer and diabetic screenings, physical fitness, and nutritional guidance. Transportation is often provided to the centers which generally function during the weekday. Nutrition centers are located in neighbor settings like a church or senior high-rise apartment or in conjunction with a senior center. They serve lunch, again, usually only on weekdays. The centers are supported by Title XX funds for those aged 60 or over. The participants pay a small fee for the meal and this is usually on a sliding-scale basis (Matteson & McConnell, 1988).

Meals-on-Wheels

Also referred to as home-delivered meals, these services provide one hot meal a day to the elderly who are confined to their home. There is usually provision for those on special diets, and some areas also provide this service on weekends and holidays. Volunteers are usually used to deliver the meals, with funding for this program being public or private.

Adult Day Care

These programs provide rehabilitative and social activities for the elderly outside the home, thereby assisting families or friends who normally care for them at home. The types of services the adult care provides can vary. Some provide daily medical care and supervision for those with chronic conditions such as stroke and Alzheimer's disease. Other day care facilities may focus on providing appropriate socialization activities. Adult day care may be a free-standing center, part of a specialized senior center, or part of a hospital setting (Crossman, 1991).

Respite Care

This is a relatively new service which can provide home care, counseling, and support groups to relieve and enrich the lives of family caregivers. Respite care can often postpone the need for institutionalization. There are four models of respite care. The home-based model uses trained sitters who provide service in the elderly person's or family's home. Sometimes the care is provided for only a few hours, overnight, a weekend, or while the family is on vacation. The second model is referred to as group day care, which is similar to adult day care previously described. Groups of elderly are provided daytime activities so that family members can run errands or just relax. Group residential care is the third model, which provides a group of elderly overnight care from one night to several weeks in a facility specially designed for respite care. The fourth model is a residential program, which provides respite care as an adjunct service, such as a nursing home or state institution which sets aside a number of beds for this purpose (Dunkle, 1991).

Hospice Care

This service is designed to provide the terminally ill the opportunity to live as fully and comfortably as possible until their death. Services provided vary according to the nature of the particular hospice. Some hospices are based within a hospital setting, but most are home-based. Elderly recipients of this care would have to be aware of their prognosis and have a life expectancy of 6 months or less. Since most hospices are home-based, a family member or a friend needs to be involved with the care. Medicare only began reimbursement for this type of service in 1984, and many argue that the reimbursement rate is too low to provide quality care (Matteson & McConnell, 1988).

The following example describes some of the problems of providing care to an individual in the community setting.

CASE EXAMPLE

Mrs. S.P. is a 98-year-old white woman who resides in a four-generational family environment. She still owns her own home, which provides her with hope and self-esteem. Her major medical problems are compressed vertebrae with arthritis and bilateral hearing loss.

Assessment Parameters for Community-based Care

1. *Environmental assessment.* Has own room in a two-story home located in the suburbs. She resides with her son's family, which includes a married granddaughter and two great-granddaughters.

2. *Activities of daily living status.* Has a home health aide who comes for 3 hours Monday through Friday. The home health aide bathes, dresses, and transfers Mrs. S.P. to a lounge chair. Mrs. S.P. no longer uses a commode but is diapered due to incontinence of bladder and bowel. She is able to feed self and spends time watching television.

3. *Mental status.* Is alert but confused at times. Has reverted back to her native tongue of Italian. Talks about going back to live in her own home.

4. *Lifestyle assessment.* Came to the United States at age 24 and worked as a domestic and waitress until married at age 27. She raised two children and assisted in the rearing of 5 grandchildren. She has been a widow since age 66, and until 5 years ago lived alone.

5. *Social support status.* Enjoys having her great-grandchildren visit, two of whom live in the same house and are constantly in and out of her room. Daughter visits 2 days a week to assist with care and provides respite for her brother. A deacon from her church visits periodically. A nurse comes once a month to assess Mrs. S.P., who at one time had a decubiti forming. Every evening Mrs. S.P. is put in a wheelchair and eats in the dining room with the rest of the family.

6. *Family status.* See previous comments.

7. *Recent life changes.* Can no longer use a walker as she claims her legs will not support her.

8. *Sensory impairment.* Vision intact, does not wear glasses, however, has significant hearing deficits in both ears. Is more sensitive to pain, which is noted when the nurse does a venipuncture for lab work.

9. Medications include Metamucil, Darvocet.

Evaluation

For the present time Mrs. S.P. is maintained in the community with a combination of informal and formal support services. There has been a great deal of mobility among the home health aides who provide care during the week. Sometimes the aides do not show and the family needs to regroup to provide coverage. On weekends and holidays there is no formal services and the family has divided up this responsibility. Mrs.

S.P. has had one hospitalization during the past year for a bladder infection. As Mrs. S.P.'s physical status continues to decline, the family may have to reconsider institutionalization.

NURSING IMPLICATIONS

Caring for the elderly is a major challenge to our society and to nursing. Institutional care continues to grow as the demand increases. In 1984, there were only 92,000 full-time registered nurses employed in nursing homes. The projections for the year 2000 range from 260,000 to one million (Ansello, 1991). Nursing homes are not the panacea for all elderly persons, but when there are not sufficient community services available or when families can no longer cope, institutionalization may be the last recourse. Home health and community-based care is a billion-dollar-a-year industry. The demand for nurses with baccalaureate and advanced degrees is projected to far exceed the supply (Jacobson, 1990). One can argue that the quality of life of an elderly person can vary with institutional versus community-based care, but the real issue is that older persons should have the right to make their own choice. In the two case examples cited, are Mrs. M.A. and Mrs. S.P. receiving the quality of life they deserve? What, if anything, could nursing do to improve these elderly women's situations?

In order for nursing to have an impact on caring for society's elderly, we first need nurses who are educated regarding issues that affect the elderly. All too often the curriculum in nursing programs excludes information on normal aging changes, psychosocial aspects of aging, and health promotion strategies with this population group. Nurses also need to be in positions where they can assist the elderly to advocate for themselves so that they can, for example, assess the services they need. Families often need the assistance of nurses to provide functional assessments and to provide appropriate counseling to handle the problems identified. It would seem important for nurses to be aware of services that their community offers so that referrals can be made.

There are two fundamental issues that affect not only policymakers, and health care providers, but also nursing (Dimond, 1989). As society moves into the next century, nurses will need to address the issue of limited resources with multiple goals. What kind of quality of life can be offered to the elderly when meeting their needs means using community funds? The second issue that involves nurses is balancing the needs of the competent with the incompetent elderly. How can we be certain that the competence levels of the elderly are judged in a fair and responsible manner?

TOPICS FOR DISCUSSION

1. Analyze your own personal feelings regarding institutionalization. Can you envision placing a family member in a nursing home? Can you envision yourself being placed in a nursing home?
2. Do you concur with Goffman that a nursing home is a total institution? Why or why not?
3. Should the current system of financing health and long-term care services for the elderly be reformed? Why?
4. Do community services for the elderly differ from those services delivered to the young?
5. How might you, as a nurse, assist families in making a decision regarding institutionalization of a family member?

REFERENCES

Ansello, E. F. (1991, February). Aging issues for the year 2000. *Caring Magazine*, *10*, 4–12.

Brody, J. A., & Foley, D. (1985). Epidemiologic considerations. In Schneider, E. L. (Ed.), *The teaching nursing home* (pp. 9–25). New York: Raven Press.

Brooke, V. (1989, March/April). How elders adjust. *Geriatric Nursing*, *10*, 66–68.

Chenitz, W. R. (1983, March/April). Entry into nursing home as status passage: A theory to guide nursing practice. *Geriatric Nursing*, *4*, 92–97.

Crossman, L. (1991). Nursing dynamics: Community care for the elderly. In W. C. Chenitz, J. T. Stone, & S. A. Salisbury (Eds.), *Clinical gerontological nursing* (pp. 589–597). Philadelphia, PA: Saunders.

Dimond, M. (1989). Health care and the aging population. *Nursing Outlook*, 37, 76–77.

Dunkle, R. E. (1988). Alternatives to institutionalization. In C. S. Kart, E. K. Metress, & S. P. Metress (Eds.), *Aging, health and society* (pp. 340–357). Boston, MA: Jones and Bartlett.

Goffman, E. (1961). *Asylums*. Garden City, NY: Doubleday.

Jacobson, J. M. (1990). Nursing's response to the aging population. *Home Healthcare Nurse*, *8*, 24–28. (May/June)

Johnson, M. A., & Werner, C. (1982, September). We had no choice: A study in familial guilt feelings surrounding nursing home care. *Journal of Gerontological Nursing*, *8*, 641–645, 654.

Kart, C. S., Metress, E. K., & Metress, S. P. (1988). *Aging, health and society*. Boston, MA: Jones and Bartlett.

Kovar, M. G., & Feinleib, M. (1991). Older Americans present a double challenge: Preventing disability and providing care. *American Journal of Public Health*, *81*, 287–288. (March)

Lamb, D. R. (1992). Many elderly see nursing homes in their future. *Report: the Official Newsletter of the New York State Nurses Association*, *23*, 7. (March)

Matteson, M. A., & McConnell, E. S. (1988). *Gerontological nursing: Concepts and Practice*. Philadelphia, PA: Saunders.

Mikhail, M. L. (1992). Psychological responses to relocation to a nursing home. *Journal of Gerontological Nursing, 18*, 35–38. (March)

Miller, L. L. (1991). Models for respite care. In W. C. Chenitz, J. T. Stone, & S. A. Salisbury (Eds.), *Clinical gerontological nursing* (pp. 599–611). Philadelphia, PA: Saunders.

Murtaugh, C. M., Kemper, P., & Spillman, B. C. (1990). The risk of nursing home use in later life. *Medical Care, 28*, 952–962. (October)

Phillips, L. R. (1989). Elder—family caregiver relationships. *Nursing Clinics of North America, 24*, 795–807. (September)

Porcino, J. (1983). *Growing older, getting better*. Reading, MA: Addison-Wesley.

Selker, L. G., & Broski, D. C. (1988). An aging society: I. Implications for health care needs. II. Impacts on allied health education and practice. *Gerontology and Geriatrics Education, 8*(3/4), 107–148.

Smallegan, M. (1985). There was nothing else to do: Need for care before nursing home admission. *Gerontologist, 25*, 364–369.

U. S. Senate Special Committee on Aging. (1984). *Aging America: Trends and projections*. Washington, DC: American Association of Retired Persons.

Zarle, N. C. (1989, September). Continuity of care: Balancing care of elders between health care settings. *Nursing Clinics of North America, 24*, 697–705.

PART III

Nursing and Society

12

Dilemmas Posed by Environmental Issues

Vern L. Bullough

Environmental issues have always been of concern to nurses. Dealing with them led to the development of community health nursing and industrial nursing early in the 20th century. These issues have also forced increasing government intervention into health care. For example, a variety of governmental units have long been engaged in assuring safe supplies of food and water, effective management of sewage and municipal wastes, the control or elimination of vector-borne illnesses, and numerous other public health measures.

Our growing awareness of the complexity of environmental issues has not made it easier to find solutions. On this issue nurses have often disagreed. This is because the piecemeal solutions which were effective in the past in dealing with specific problems no longer seem adequate, and more drastic action seems to be required. The question is further complicated by a major disagreement over major causal factors.

Nowhere was this more evident than at the first Earth Summit Conference held in Rio de Janeiro in June 1992, a conference in which delegates from most of the countries of the world participated. Delegates seem to have divided into two different and conflicting camps in the way they conceptualized the basic problem. It was only by recognizing that both conceptions led to the same result—that the world's resources were limited—and that certain activities put the environment under greater stress than others—that any agreements could be made. Part of the difficulty is that ultimate solutions, regardless of the causal factors, have the potential to drastically change our lifestyles.

One side in the environmental conflict claims the problem is essentially one of overpopulation; that the growing demands of an ever-increasing population are straining the earth's resources simply to feed and house people. The statistics are scary. According to the United Nations, the world's population will increase to 13 billion by the end of the 21st century, or two and a half times its present size (*Newsweek*, June 1, 1992). Since more people are now living in the world than ever lived in all the times past, the insults to the environment which now exist can only escalate. If consumption grows at just two-thirds the rate of the past 25 years, it would quadruple in 70 years; in the year 2100, by these modest projections, the world would need to be producing 20 times as much as it is today. Few believe that goal is fully realizable and the inevitable result will be overcultivation, soil exhaustion, destruction of nature, and widespread famine. Some, like Garret Hardin (1993), a founder of human ecology, have compared the situation to a lifeboat which is as full as it can get as it departs from the sinking ship; to take on even one more passenger swimming around in the water will capsize the boat and kill everyone. The more extreme advocates of this view hold that the only possible solution for those on the lifeboat is to prevent any others from coming aboard. In terms of public policy they would argue that since the inevitable result of overpopulation will be famine, starvation, and misery for everyone, anything done to alleviate the suffering will only aggravate the ultimate problem, and so we have to ignore the suffering of others and concentrate on our own survival. More moderate advocates of this view feel that it might be possible to trail a rope behind the lifeboat onto which some might grasp until something better turned up. They advocate the importance of limiting population through various forms of birth control; of introducing new techniques in agriculture which put less stress on the environment; and of the development of nonpolluting industry to help support such populations, but hold that this policy can only be successful in the long run if the world population explosion is slowed down and a stable population is achieved.

In a sense, this more extreme view is a continuation of the views of Thomas Malthus, who in the 18th century first argued that the world was outgaining its food supply as food supplies grew only in an arithmetic ratio (1, 2, 3, 4) wheras population grew in a geometric ratio (1, 2, 4, 8). Malthus went on to claim that the inevitable result would be ever-greater human misery for masses of people. Critics of the Malthusian view argue that people have been decrying overpopulation for the past two centuries but somehow the world has survived. The nature of the argument has changed, however, because now the problem is not visualized simply as the inability of the food supply to keep up with population, but the exhaustion of the world's resources, ranging from the rain forests to the decline in numbers of animal and plant diversity caused by the growing population. It was the danger to the environment posed by greater populations that caused Garret Hardin to put forth the concept of the overloaded lifeboat. When such a view is pushed to extreme, it is an argument for total selfishness, and a justification for those who have it made, to ignore the problems of the poor, the weak, and the ill.

The opposite view of causation to that of overpopulation is that the basic environmental problems are caused by overconsumption, and not overpopulation. This is the view put forth by many of the Third World countries, as well as by many environmentalists in the United States. Advocates of this view point out that countries like the United States consume a disproportionate share of the world's food and products, and that it is our conspicuous waste from households and industry that are the main causes of the world' environmental crisis. They also argue that Americans tend to accuse others for doing what they themselves have already done. The United States, for example, has consumed all but 5% of its virgin timber, and yet countries like Brazil point out that it is the Americans who lead the criticism of Brazil's destruction of the Amazonian rain forests. It is our overconsumption, our vast demand for fuel-inefficient automobiles, and the emission of hydrocarbons into the atmosphere which many claim are the main causes of the environmental crisis. The issue is further complicated by the attempts of other countries to match our consumption patterns, a competition which has escalated the crisis of the environment. The solution, for advocates of this view, is to cut down on the products of affluence: cars, gadgets, luxury yachts, and what-have-you, and give more of the resources to the poor and hungry of the world. The poor countries want royalties and property rights as compensation for, among other things, supplying pharmaceutical companies with their genetic treasures; for protecting their rain forests, which affect the climate for everyone; and for cutting down on their inefficient polluting industries.

The nub of the problem is that advocates of this view hold that it is not enough for the richer countries to give subsidies to the poorer ones. The richer ones must also emphasize the potential of biodiversity in their own countries—curtailing the cutting of Oregon virgin timber, for example, to save the spotted owl. At the Rio conference, where the participants eventually agreed that strong action was needed on the major concerns both of overpopulation and overconsumption, then President George Bush refused to sign the treaty on biodiversity because it might endanger employment opportunities in the United States. He argued that much more research is needed before any conclusions can be drawn or effective political action taken. With such an attitude expressed by the American president, it is no wonder that the world itself has difficulty in coming to terms with the environmental dangers to health and welfare. There are simply no easy answers.

There is still a third issue connected with the environment that is just beginning to emerge, namely the association between the destruction of environment and the appearance of new diseases. It is evident that in recent years a whole series of new diseases have appeared, the most notable of which is AIDS, but others include Ebola, Marburg, and yellow fever viruses that probably first appeared in monkeys, and the Rift Valley virus, originally diagnosed in cattle, sheep, and mosquitoes. In the United States recent years have seen the appearance of the Hanta virus in the Southwest, the tick-born Lyme disease in the Northeast, and the virus that causes dengue fever almost everywhere.

Some epidemiologists have theorized that the appearance of these new killers are due to devastation of the environment, especially intrusions of humans into new ecological settings, such as the rain forests that allow previously isolated viruses and infectious microbes to spread rapidly to large numbers of people. They argue that the diseases have always existed but only in limited areas and infected only limited populations and the very isolation stopped them from spreading.

One of the best illustrations of this theory is the case of the nonfatal Oropouche virus in Brazil, which appeared in 1960 and soon after caused a flu-like epidemic among 11,000 people who suffered from high fevers, headaches, and muscle aches. After some 19 years of epidemiological research it was found that the virus was spread by forest-dwelling midges in Brazil and when the forests were cleared and cacao (the source of chocolate) was planted the midges did not disappear but instead found a new, even more ideal breeding ground in the discarded hulls of cacao beans.

Similar factors might be behind the emergence of AIDS and the other "new" diseases although the complete answer is as yet uncertain. There is, however, enough evidence that radical changes in environment pose new disease potential that a panel of infectious disease experts produced a report holding that "environmental changes probably account for most emerging diseases." Not everyone agrees and the evidence is still fragmentary (Gibbons, 1993). Still, what this kind of research emphasizes is that environmental issues have the potential to confront nurses in almost every aspect of nursing care.

It is not only new diseases that might come from destruction of the environment, but many other traditional diseases are also affected by the environmental factors. The influence of such environmental factors might well be a major reason why modern medicine and the health care system in general has failed to make a significant impact on some of the modern epidemics, such as cancer. Everyone knows that cancer has environmental causes and the American public has been flooded by a constant flow of warnings about the danger of air pollution, contamination of drinking supplies, carcinogenic effects of food additives, PCBs, asbestos, vinyl chlorides, pesticides, saccharine, and many more things we ingest, breathe, or come in contact with.Because there is ongoing debate about the threshold limit values of some of the carcinogens, and the validity of animal research application to humans is not always clear, experts can disagree on causal factors. Still it is clear that all of us are continually being exposed to a multitude of disease-causing factors.

The question is how far we should go in attempting to redirect traditional American practices in order to lessen the dangers of environmental pollution. On the one hand there has been a rapid growth in government legislation and agencies putting limits on what corporations can do. Such legislation has been effective. A good example is the Federal Coalminer Safety Act of 1969 and the Occupation Safety and Health Act (OSHA) of 1970, both of which led to a drastic reduction of environmental hazards encountered on the job. It has been estimated that the enforcement of OSHA, for example, led to at least a 20% decline in industrial accidents between its enactment, in 1970, and 1978, and the rates have continued to decline (National Safety Council, 1987). The Environmental Protection Agency (EPA) established in 1976 has also led to investigations of chemicals and toxic substances that represent unreasonable risks to the environment and has forced elimination of many of the most toxic substances. Each of these acts was opposed by many in industry because their enforcement resulted in higher production costs; they were also often opposed by labor groups who feared they would cut employment, and by consumer groups because the end result might be higher prices. These fears were real enough and in a sense might be said to have been justified, one reason for the flight of American industry to plants along the Mexican border is the lack of the costs of observing environmental safeguards which are almost nonexistent in many Third World countries. Some of the effects of this neglect are listed in the chapter by Patricia Castiglia elsewhere in this book. At the same time, this flight of industry from United States has led to a drop in real wages and an increase in unemployment.

This emphasizes the dilemma in which we find ourselves. The problem is not just with industry, however, but with ourselves. Victor Fuchs (1974), while recognizing environmental factors as very important, went on to assert that

> [the] greatest potential for reducing coronary disease, cancer, and other major killer still lies in altering personal behavior. (pp. 26, 46)

Put simply, we are overconsuming things that pose environmental danger to each of us. The question then becomes just how far we should go in putting limits on individual freedom. We know, for example, that smoking has a strong correlation with cancer. Though the government has ordered cigarette companies to put warnings on their packs of cigarettes and levied ever heavier taxes on tobacco products, smoking does not just affect the health of the individual who smokes, but others as well who do not smoke. Should the government ban cigarettes entirely? The government once prohibited the sale of alcoholic beverages, a policy that was later voted out. Would a ban on tobacco prove any more effective?

The issue becomes even more complex when we realize that the problem of overconsumption, in this case of tobacco products, is an economic burden to all of us. This is because the costs of care for the person who gets cancer or suffers from heart disease or any of the numerous other ailments now attributed to tobacco, costs each of us tax money, since long-term care for many of those so afflicted is paid for through Medicare, Medicaid, or other public money. Even if treatment is paid for through private insurance funds, it raises the cost of our medical insurance, whether it is paid for by the government or privately sponsored. Our whole system of health care is based upon what might be called the nofault principle, that regardless of whether we might have taken actions which caused our disease or illness, we are not at fault. Yet some people are certainly more at fault than others.

Any number of diseases can be attributed to overconsumption or, in individual terms, overindulgence, whether it be due to alcoholism, reckless driving, lack of sexual control, or even eating. Many of the more expensive foods, such as meats, are high in chloresterol which has been associated with atherosclerosis. Overconsumption or overindulgence leads to a greater amount of waste material, and the more well-to-do use far more materials, whether it be food, gasoline, or lumber, than do the poor.

The American scene also offers examples of the problems of overpopulation, particularly if overpopulation is associated with the inability of people to care adequately for their families or children. Just as we can equate overconsumption to overindulgence, so can overpopulation be equated with poverty. Poverty poses different environmental health problems than exist among the more well-to-do, since it is the richer who are producing the pollutants which affect the poor. Housing in poorer neighborhoods is often older and more dilapidated and contains some of the contaminants which earlier generations did not realize were so dangerous, such as lead-based paint or asbestos insulation. It is the poor who are less able to escape from the harm of the polluted environment, who are more likely to live by dump sites, and who are the most susceptible to environmental toxins.

One of the early studies of lead poisoning published in 1966 described a so-called lead belt that consisted primarily of poor urban areas in the East and Midwest. The authors found that 20 to 40% of the children in these areas had elevated lead levels, primarily from ingestion of paint chips or other lead-contaminated products. As a result of such findings, Congress in 1971 enacted the Lead Prevention Act, which allocated funds for the establishment of screening facilities under the direction of the Surgeon General and the removal of lead paints from dwelling in poor areas, as well as prohibiting any use of lead additives to paint manufactured in the future. In spite of such actions, however, clean-up procedures have been slow and lead poisoning in children ingesting lead chips remains a major problem. Lead often appears in solder which connects pipes that carry our drinking water; many of the toy soldiers, miniature cars, and molded utensils of the past also contain lead, as do pottery glazes and gunpowder. All of these sources of lead are being eliminated, as was one of the major sources of lead poisoning, the lead in gasoline. Still, lead remains a danger. Chronic lead exposure occurs most frequently among children younger than 5 years of age. Children who exhibit symptoms such as fatigue, pallor, appetite loss, irritability, sleep disturbances, and even behavior change may have been ingesting lead for months. The first areas to sustain damage are the pathways of heme (the iron proptoprophyrin constituent of hemoglobin), and then the kidney and liver. Prolonged high level exposure results in nerve damage caused by the degeneration of the axons and demyelination of the peripheral nerves. The problems is complicated because diets poor in calcium, phosphorus, and iron, result in greater absorption of lead by the body (Leopard & Bullough, 1990).

In fact, whatever mineral or metal toxicants there are, from arsenic to asbestos, the poor are more likely to suffer from their aftereffects, unless the source of the contaminants is in the workplace. The poor are also more likely to live in areas where industrial pollutants are the greatest, where garbage and refuse are least likely to be picked up, where housing is the oldest, and to drive the older, more gas-guzzling automobiles. They have higher infant mortality rates, lower rates of educational achievement, poorer nutrition, and lower rates of longevity. Again, some low-income individuals have less adequate diets than others because of the way they choose to spend resources. Even individuals on general public assistance or food assistance programs feel that they, and not the health professionals, have the right to choose the kind of food they eat.

This raises the same kind of control questions potential in all issues of environment. Should the poverty patient and client be encouraged to eat better by being offered only the more healthy foods and actively discouraged from eating or drinking of other foods and liquids? How far should we go in encouraging them to use some form of birth control, when it is clear that many families cannot adequately support even themselves?

These kind of questions are actually being posed and answered in other areas of the world. For example, China, which now has a population of over 1 billion, was slow in awakening to the dangers of overpopulation and only did so in the early 1980s. Chinese officials now feel that the dangers of overpopulation are holding back their development and pushing their resources to the limit. The solution which China adopted in the 1980s and which continues in force is to establish the one-child family, not only as an ideal but by legal fiat.

In order for a Chinese couple to consider having a child, they need to get a permit from the authorities to try to get pregnant. If the permit is granted, they then have a period of time in which they can get pregnant; if they fail to do so their quota is assigned to another person. To prevent individuals from getting pregnant without the proper permit, the Chinese danwei, a governmental unit to which all urban Chinese belong, and similar to a rural commune, enforces the requirement. Specific women in the danwei are designated to perform monthly inspections on all women in their childbearing years. If any woman has missed a period or there are other indications of possible pregnancy and the couple do not have the certificate allowing pregnancy, they are required to go through an abortion. Once a couple has a child, the woman is encouraged to become sterilized by giving the existing child special advantages for schooling and even monetary rewards to the family. Some couples manage to have more than one child in spite of the attempts at enforcement, particularly those living in rural areas where such enforcement is more lax. When this occurs, the parents can be fined, lose their jobs, and even in extreme cases have their children taken from them. Some individuals and groups, however, particularly some of the ethnic minorities, are exempt from the one-child family limits. The requirements for exemptions are set out by the government and enforced by the danwei authorities. As of this writing, the policy still remains in effect, although the government has shown increasing willingness to make exceptions, particularly for those families whose first (and therefore only child) was a girl. One reason for the willingness to grant exceptions was the recognition by the government of widespread infanticide of girl babies.

This policy seems extreme to almost all Americans and one that no American would adopt. Instead, we encourage families to plan their family size by making the various methods of birth control or abortion alternative available, and giving women greater and greater opportunities in the workplace. The result has been a drop in American family size. But what if this is not enough? Some countries in which there is consider-able opposition to artificial means of contraception, have culturally adapted to limiting families in other ways. In Ireland, for example, late marriage of both men and women and celibacy, at least for the women, until marriage has served to cut down the birth rate. Other countries have followed different patterns, but it is primarily the underdeveloped coun-tries, where children are seen as old-age insurance, where the birth rate remains high.

Though we are plagued with poverty on the one hand, we are the larg-est per capita consumers of material goods in the world on the other. Do we ignore such problems or do we take preventative steps to solve some of them? Certainly we cannot ask the rest of the world to do what we cannot do for ourselves. The problem is that almost any action we take, except for massive education policies, will imply greater interference in our personal life-styles.

The U. S. Public Health Service in its report, *Healthy People 2000: National Health Promotion and Disease Prevention Objectives* (1990) listed a number of environmental health objectives, few of which can be met without some form of governmental action. These include reduction of exposure to toxic agents and contaminants; improving the supplies of safe drinking water; lowering the existence of lead-based paint in older homes; encouraging the use of recyclable materials; tracking and defin-ing environmental diseases; reducing exposure to tobacco smoking; improving occupational safety and health; lowering the rate of cancer deaths; improving maternal and infant health; lessening the incidence of diabetes and chronic disabling conditions; and increasing the use and dissemination of effective contraceptives.

Such a policy implies attempts to lessen the consequences of poverty by providing better social services and educational facilities, and work-ing to establish a minimum living standard. It does not, however, address the problem of overconsumption. Obviously one way to do so would be to put a high tax on the so-called luxuries, put a limitation on the num-ber of product choices available, and charge more for excessive waste, all of which would probably only make a greater differential between the rich and the poor in this country since it would limit the choices of the poor more than the rich.

There are really no easy decisions in dealing with the environment. The author himself is ambivalent about which possible solutions to adopt, but it seems clear that the issues will increasingly dominate the political area. As nurses we will be called upon to make recommendations and to voice our opinions. Hopefully we can do so with some understanding of what the issues are. Though each of us can adjust our own personal life-style to one we feel is environmentally sound, we also have to think about what limitations, if any, we want to put on others. For any policy to be effective, nurses will have a leadership role in education.

TOPICS FOR DISCUSSION

1. One issue is the whole concept of the overcrowded lifeboat. If this view is widely adopted, what would its effect be on nurses and nursing care? If resources are limited, should each patient be treated the same, or should resources be concentrated on those who potentially have the most to contribute to society? Does altruism have a place?
2. Does a government, such as China, have the right to put limits on the number of children an individual can have? What would you do if you lived in China and either you or your wife found yourself pregnant a second time?
3. If curtailing the lumber industry to save the habitat of the spotted owl is necessary but would also lead to unemployment, what policy would you advocate?
4. Since second-hand smoke from tobacco users is believed to be dangerous for those who inhale it, what rights do smokers have? Do nurses have a special obligation to society to set an example in this regard?
5. Should the state or local government pay to repaint old houses that are covered inside and out with lead-based paint?
6. Which governmental action would you advocate to address the problem of overconsumption?

REFERENCES

Bullough, B., & Rosen, G. (1992). *Preventive medicine in the United States: 1900–1990.* Canton, MA: Science History.

Fuchs, V. (1974). *Who shall live? Health, economics, and social choice.* New York: Basic Books.

Harzdin, G. (1993). *Ecology, economics, and population taboos.* New York: Oxford University Press.

Leopard, M., & Bullough, V. (1990). "Environmental issues. In B. Bullough & V. Bullough (Eds.), *Nursing in the community* (pp. 129–145). St. Louis: Mosby.

National Safety Council. (1987). *Work injury and illness rates.* Chicago: Author.

Newsweek. (1992, June 15). Why Rio will make history (p. 33).

U.S. Public Health Service. *Healthy People 2000: National Health Promotion and Disease Prevention Objectives.* (1992). (DHHHS Publication No. (PHS) 91–50212). Washington DC: Superintendent of Documents.

13

Nursing Care in a Culturally Diverse Nation

Marilyn Hyche Johnson

As the United States moves toward the 21st century, our nation is becoming more culturally, racially, and ethnically diverse. It is predicted that African-American, Asian-American, Hispanic-American, and Native-American population groups when combined will comprise the numerical majority by the middle of the next century. While there is some disagreement over the potential size of these groups, we do know that our immigrant and indigenous minority populations are growing at a faster rate than our majority population. These groups, like the previous waves of immigrants and migrants, are seeking the "American dream" of a better life for themselves and their families. Many will need and seek health care and will become users of our health care systems. Generally, in terms of health, culturally diverse groups from geographic areas outside of Europe, excluding Asians, have not fared well. Health care for members of nondominant cultural groups has typically been poorer in quality than that afforded members of the dominant American culture. There are disparities not only in quality of care, but in accessibility to care and in illness outcomes (U.S. Department of Commerce, 1991).

Are we prepared to provide optimum care for these groups of culturally diverse people? Unless we are prepared to drastically alter our existing approach to health care for these groups, the answer is, unfortunately, no. Currently, the American health care delivery system is grounded in a monocultural, scientific model. The white middle-class male is the archetype of the monocultural model. And the approaches, research, and treatments that work for him will not necessarily work for women, children, and people of color. Weidman (1979) argued that scientific or modern medicine operates on the assumption that in matters of health, only scientific knowledge is valid. The modern health care delivery system has obtained a legally sanctioned status and concomitant prerogatives which allow it to generally disregard the health beliefs and customary health behaviors of its clients. This represents a serious error from a humanistic point of view. It also presents a monumental problem for culturally diverse clients, first by undermining their own belief system and meaning structure, and second, by asking them to accept instantly and without question the value, complexity, and meanings of this superior scientific medical system. In the end, the goal of maintaining optimum health is lost when the monocultural health care system interacts with the culturally diverse client without accommodating his/her culture.

Kluckhohn (1976) suggested that the monocultural value system within which nurses are educated in the United States tends to render them future-oriented, individualistic in decision making, professionally action-oriented, and believers in the controllability of illness. When the client shares the same values as the nurse, interaction goes well. Problems occur when there are value or cultural divergences.

Weidman (1979) projected that when a monocultural system like ours interacts with people from other cultures, the following three predictable outcomes occur: first, an absence of improved health status; second, a difference between clients' and health care providers' cultural orientations focus them on different problems; and finally, intolerance, frustration, and possibly contempt for the client's cultural style emerge when it was out of synchronization with the dominant medical perspective.

THE IMPORTANCE OF CULTURAL DIVERSITY

A major reason cultural diversity is so important to nursing is the fact that nurses have more direct interaction with clients than do any other members of the health team. Therefore, as clients become increasingly more culturally diverse, it becomes vital that nurses become sensitive to and knowledgeable about cultural aspects of nursing care.

To give meaningful and competent nursing care, the nurse must have an understanding of the client's lifestyle, health and illness beliefs, his/her traditional and professional care practices, world view, ethics, and values. Nurses need to understand their own culture and how and where it intersects and deviates from that of their clients. While the concept of transcultural nursing has been around for a number of years, it has not become the norm for most nursing education programs or nursing practice settings. Even as I argue for the need for the integration of transcultural nursing in all nursing curricula, I recognize that there are nurses who believe that nursing can and has delivered competent care without special sensitivity to cultural knowledge. These nurses tend to resist the addition of transcultural nursing content to nursing curricula and to clinical practice settings because they believe that nursing is complex and multidimensional enough. Further, they argue that short hospital stays require shorter, more focused assessments. What they fail to consider are the challenges to competent and meaningful health care provision fostered by the cultural uniqueness of each client population. In addition, there is evidence to suggest that these nurses have failed to recognize the problems nurses cause when they impose their culture on clients from other cultural backgrounds.

CULTURAL TERMS DEFINED

Cultural imposition occurs when the dominant culture practices ethnocentrism, defined as a belief in the inherent superiority of one's own group and culture accompanied by a feeling of contempt for other groups and cultures. Numerous problems develop as a result of our ethnocentricity. These problems range from a lack of meaningful communication and understanding to uninformed decision making, conflicting values, and insensitive responses to inadequate health care. One cannot treat the whole person without knowledge of that person. One way to promote health is to understand what each person brings with them. Each of us may view the same situation very differently because of our level of education, income, where we come from, what we do, our politics, our religion, our race or ethnicity, and our values and beliefs. Thus, what one person sees and how that vision affects him or her is often unique. Uniqueness or difference is to be interpreted neither as inferior nor incorrect, only as different. We must respect other people's experiences and understand how these experiences might lead them to interpret situations they encounter in ways that are meaningful to them from a different world view.

Cultural imposition is an outcome of the ethnocentrism and racism that permeate American culture and its social institutions. Ethnocentrism and racism are so pervasive that they are often considered neutral, and normal, escaping notice and scrutiny. Very few, if any, people growing up in this culture develop without being affected, socialized, and conditioned by their influence. In the long run, it has a negative impact on all Americans. The 1980s witnessed a time of growing ethnocentrism, a withdrawal from previous governmental and social positions on equality, and increasing ethnic and racial tensions. The recent Rodney King beating by Los Angeles policemen, the subsequent trial and acquittal, and the resulting anger and violence has left many Americans angry, fearful, and silent.

Many people avoid discussing cultural and racial differences due to their feelings of anger and frustration or from fear of saying the wrong thing, or of saying what is really on their minds or being labelled a racist or prejudiced. We must, however, face each other and talk about cultural differences, racism, and ethnocentrism in order to change, grow, and improve. Our very discomfort in discussing our social "isms" is a symptom of the problem.

Two other terms in need of definition are racism and prejudice. Racism may be defined as "any attitude, action, or institutional structure which subordinates a person or group because of their color" (U.S. Commission on Civil Rights, 1970). Racism is different from racial prejudice or discrimination because it involves having the power to carry out systematic discriminatory practices through the major institutions of our society, namely our political, judicial, educational, and economic institutions. Prejudice, on the other hand, is a preconceived judgement or opinion usually denoting an individual attitude of antipathy or active hostility against another social group, usually racially defined (Abercrombie, Hill, & Turner, 1984).

WHAT NURSING EDUCATION CAN DO

Nursing students need to be aware of these terms and their own feelings, beliefs, and thoughts about them. Faculty can facilitate student awareness by encouraging them to discuss the terms and issues, share experiences, and write down their feelings, concerns, fears, and doubts. It is important for nursing education to address the sensitive issues of race and culture and not devalue them, they are integral to understanding the client, and will not go away. Ignoring them makes nurses less able to provide appropriate culturally sensitive care for diverse clients. Schools of nursing must teach students to physically assess people of color, and to socially and culturally assess all clients. In preparing for the next century, it will be crucial to prepare nurses to become sensitive to the untoward health effects of living with anger, frustration, injustice, inequality, poverty, and environmental hazards. Learning how these conditions of living are manifested in the health status and the type of illnesses culturally diverse populations are prone to is extremely germane to improving their care. It is important to discuss why some people gain access to treatment while others with the same conditions do not. It is necessary to know the relationship between hopelessness, economic deprivation, nutrition, education, and quality of health, as well as the type of health care delivered.

Culture determines how people decide and perceive that they are ill and how, where, and when they seek treatment for their symptoms. Nurses have recognized that during crisis, some culturally diverse clients revert to their native language and traditional health practices. Now they must recognize which of the traditional sources of care and/or folk medical practices utilized by culturally diverse clients have the potential to interact positively, neutrally, or negatively with modern Western medical practices.

The major problem experienced by nurses in all health care delivery systems is likely to be a function of their relationship to their clients. All too often, nurses have been prepared to expect to care for a certain type of client. It is within the monocultural context that nurses envision the ideal client upon whom they base their interventions and their expectations. When the actual client does not match up with the preconceived client envisioned by the nurse, frustration, conflict, and problems often ensue. When nurses practice in urban settings, they typically meet a more socially, ethnically, racially, economically, and religiously differentiated population. Since these diverse clients tend to be much further from the ideal, nurses, unsure of the best approach, frequently treat them as if they were ideal, and end up frustrated with the client's response. Or, recognizing their difference, the nurse may treat them according to their cultural descriptions and end up frustrated again.

The following example of treating a culturally diverse client as ideal occurred when a student, having learned that clients have a right to know about their condition and are interested in participating in their care, made an assumption about her client. The nurse gave her twenty-year-old female Mexican-American client frank, but brief, information about her disease and asked her to make decisions about her care. Assuming that the client's quiet, compliant response indicated agreement, the nurse initiated the treatment plan. Shortly thereafter, she became frustrated when the client did not comply with her plan. In fact, deference to authority, both in family to elder and male members and in health care settings to doctors and nurses, and valuing politeness and courtesy are characteristics of Mexican-Americans that Anthony-Tkach (1981) suggests nurses need to be aware of. Had the student prior knowledge of these cultural characteristics, frustration could have been avoided by exploring expectations of care, degree of desired participation, and inclusion of family members with her client.

Conversely, in another situation, a nurse familiar with Micronesian cultural values was aware that many of them viewed ample body fat as evidence of economic success and caring by their families. Based on this information, the nurse decided that it would be useless to discuss weight loss and diet with her overweight client diagnosed with arterio sclerotic heart disease. In this example, the nurse's knowledge confounded her approach to the client, causing her to make an inappropriate decision and end up feeling frustrated. The culturally astute nurse assesses the individual and develops a plan of care that is congruent with the client's own values, beliefs, and health care practices, and uses her advocacy role for clients and families who have not adopted the modern health care role of the autonomous and self-directed client.

What is needed is a new vision of the possible client you may serve and some knowledge of their differences, as well as the best approaches to achieve optimum health care in spite of or because of those differences. It is here that the cultural descriptions of various cultural groups developed by various nurse researchers (Bodner & Leininger, 1992; Bullough & Bullough, 1982; Davis, 1992; Giger, Davidhizar & Turner, 1992; Leininger, 1991a; Saylor & Taylor, 1993) become invaluable. The first thing the health provider must do is to understand difference and fight the seemingly automatic process of equating difference with inferiority or deficiency. Next, nurses must recognize their own ethnocentric attitudes, beliefs, and behaviors, and recognize that the modern health care delivery system ignores the traditional or folk care system. In this way, wittingly or unwittingly, health professionals communicate to culturally diverse clients that their perceptions, knowledge, and experience have little significance, that their beliefs are not worth inquiring about, and that their customary health practices and traditions are to be disregarded (Weidman, 1979).

Nurses must become more sensitive to and begin to appreciate and value differences. To this end, it is helpful to envision American society more appropriately as a salad bowl instead of as a melting pot. In a salad, each ingredient is distinct, bringing its own uniqueness to the whole; whereas the melting pot paradigm requires people to give up their uniqueness and blend together to form something different. Although it is usual to hear people preach tolerance, remember that tolerance implies putting up with someone or permitting something you would not naturally endure. Tolerating culturally diverse individuals or groups that are generally unworthy of your attention is viewed by them as condescending and degrading. People want to be accepted, or at least respected, not merely tolerated.

It is also important for nurses to recognize that racial and ethnic minorities in this country are no more monolithic than majority populations. They vary from each other according to many factors, among them education, experiences, maturity, socio economic status, where and how they were socialized, values, and so on.

A general principle in relating with people from diverse cultures is to remember that we are all more alike than different. Most people want the same things out of life: health, comfort, home, family, freedom, justice, happiness, success for their children. We all belong to one race, the human race. Society in general and health care professionals in particular must get beyond the artificial racial and ethnic distinctions they have been socialized to see and react to. For example, simply labeling a client as Black, White, or Hispanic fails to prepare the nurse to identify whether that individual's ethnic or national orientation is Canadian, Nigerian, American, Puerto Rican, Jamaican, or Mexican. Racial categories are not very helpful. Knowing a person's culture, values, and experiences provides better clues to understanding.

In the past, colleges and universities have been profoundly negligent in their inherent role of intellectual leadership. Rather than challenge the widespread assumptions about race and ethnicity, scholars have at times muddled the issue, and thus, adding to the confusion, pursued idiosyncratic research, and/or become bogged down in circular debate. Research on expectation and perception has demonstrated that people often form highly developed impressions of others from rather limited information. Information that has been particularly salient in forming social perceptions is race and social class. In the future, colleges and universities could better prepare health care practitioners by requiring faculty and students to systematically examine their beliefs and behaviors in relation to culturally different groups; unlearn false beliefs; and identify their biases and prejudices, but most importantly, recognize that knowledge is not neutral. Knowledge, culturally determined and validated, has meaning in a cultural context and, thus, is not universally applicable.

Various researchers have studied diverse cultural groups and provided descriptions, explanations and general facts about specific cultures that have expanded the growth of transcultural knowledge (Axtell, 1991; Galanti, 1991; Platt & Persico, 1992; Rosenthal & Frenkel, 1992; Spector, 1991). Schools of nursing should introduce transcultural nursing concepts early in the curriculum, and then help students learn about health beliefs of the clients most frequently encountered in their clinical agencies and geographic region. Cultural research studies help nurses immensely to gain understanding of culturally diverse clients. The danger, however, is that these cultural descriptions may be taken concretely to describe all people from a specific culture, and/or applied without additional assessment and decision-making. In addition, greater cultural information has the capacity to inadvertently permit more sophisticated stereotypes.

Another way to better understand and integrate cultural concepts is for nursing as a profession to open itself up to more ethnic, racial, and gender diversity. Nursing needs more minority clinical practitioners, faculty, and administrators. The current under representation of minorities in the health care professions, meaning that their rate of participation as health care providers is less than their percent of population, is expected to continue or increase in the next century, while, at the same time, the health care needs of minority clients are projected to increase.

If nursing fails to take action to better meet the needs of this growing culturally diverse population, it is conceivable that these groups could mobilize themselves to demand and lobby for changes in health care practices. The result could be the imposition of nursing care approaches from outside the nursing profession. For example, nursing education institutions and practice settings could identify or be forced to develop general guidelines and formalized routine steps to the care of culturally diverse clients and require nurses to adopt those standards of behavior. A system of reward and punishment could be developed to ensure compliance, regardless of the nurses's feelings and attitude toward the client. While this is not a preferred method for integrating cultural concepts, as nursing becomes increasingly regulated, it is conceivable. It is likely that this approach would be grounded in the fact that you can change and control people's behavior much easier than you can change their attitude and opinions. The trend has been established that society and government will not wait for professionals to decide when to more adequately meet the needs of their constituents. And the constituency of culturally diverse clients is projected to constitute over 50% of the total U.S. population by the year 2050 (Ross-Gordon, Martin, & Briscoe, 1990). In a pluralistic democracy, nursing must recognize diversity as a basis for unity.

FOSTERING CULTURAL SENSITIVITY

Cultural sensitivity precedes cultural competence. Most of us are aware of people who are different; cultural sensitivity in this instance means awareness of difference, how it developed, and what it means to that individual or group. Awareness, knowledge, and understanding are prerequisites to cultural competence.

There are numerous strategies for developing cultural awareness and sensitivity. The following 10 beginning steps are suggestions to facilitate this process.

   1. The first and most critical strategy is for nursing leaders and administrators, faculty, and staff members, to become aware of the under representation of racial, ethnic, and gender-diverse populations in nursing and to commit to cultural diversity as a goal. When you make something a goal, you are more likely to establish the necessary objectives to meet it.

2. After goal setting, the next most significant step is to establish ground rules to facilitate the development of cultural sensitivity. Participants must agree to avoid labeling, maintain confidentiality, listen, and use less value-laden and more neutral language while trying to be open, honest and nonjudgmental.

3. The nurse develops cultural sensitivity by focusing on her/his own culture first. It is important to be able to describe your own beliefs, norms, values, and world view and to recognize how your cultural identity affects your relationships with and opinions of others.

4. Treat the culturally diverse person as an individual and not as a group. This is critical to delivering individualized, competent care, but may be difficult, both because we have learned to file similar ideas, things, and persons together in our memory banks, and because every individual is born and socialized into a group.

5. Gain awareness of your nonverbal language and the manner in which it affects your interactions with people from diverse cultures, as well as your perceptions of the nonverbal behavior of others and its impact on you. Role-play various behaviors you associate with people of specific cultures with an observer or a video recorder.

6. Identify various ways to bridge differences in race, ethnicity, age, religious, sexual preference, and gender by brainstorming, group discussion, term papers, case studies, or role playing.

7. Assign a student, where possible, to a staff member of the same culture as the client in order for the student to observe and assist in the care delivery to a culturally different client. One difficulty in implementing this suggestion is the paucity of racial, ethnic, and gender-diverse nurses.

8. Hire cultural consultants to sensitize nursing faculty and staff and facilitate the development of cultural competence. Education, in the form of inservice programs, workshops and conferences, on cultural diversity, is helpful to introduce and expand cultural knowledge.

9. Foster students' reasoning and problemsolving skills by examining issues, asking why most culturally diverse groups are not a part of the mainstream and/or what impact of environmental, sociocultural, psychological, and economic factors have on health and illness and health delivery.

10. Teach students to analyze and critique existing health care delivery systems and health/illness research and identify their relevance to culturally diverse clients.

CONCLUSION

In summary, a complete assessment of cultural aspects of a client's lifestyle, health beliefs, and health practices will enhance the nurses's decision making and judgement when providing care. Nursing interventions that are sensitive and culturally relevant to the client markedly reduce the possibility of stress and conflict arising from cultural misunderstanding. This reduction of cultural misunderstanding is facilitated when the nurse has been sensitized to her own cultural biases and behaviors, as well as to those of the client.

What is judged and valued as "good" care is culturally determined, culturally based, and culturally validated. Thus, the recipient of health care from a particular cultural group can identify and define "good care" in a manner that the health care provider from another cultural group can not. Client satisfaction and cooperation with the treatment plan is related to the degree to which expectations are shared and met.

I believe that it is not possible to give competent, thorough, relevant, and satisfying nursing care to all of our clients without cultural knowledge. Dr. Madeleine Leininger (1991a, 1991b), the developer of transcultural nursing care theory in the 1960s, predicts that by the turn of the century, transcultural nursing will be a required area of preparation for all professional nursing. By that time, Leininger believes, nursing will have recognized that without a transcultural approach, the provision of knowledgeable and competent care to the diverse populations of the United States will be impossible. Nursing has the ability and the responsibility to more fully integrate culture into its education and practice, largely because the unifying and essential theme of nursing is caring. And caring for the human race must guide nursing's professional thoughts and behaviors.

TOPICS FOR DISCUSSION

1. Describe your own cultural heritage and beliefs as they relate to issues that might interfere with your feelings of acceptance in a hospital in another country. Take, for example, Japan, Egypt, or Mexico.
2. American beliefs in a slender physique are not the same as the beliefs of all other people. Explain some of the other beliefs about desirable body shape.
3. The author suggests that a salad bowl may be a better metaphor for us to consider than a melting pot. What are the implications of this other metaphor.
4. After you have learned all you can about another culture you might

find that your patient does not accept the norms of that culture, and seems to be completely Americanized. How do you deal with that situation.

REFERENCES

Abercrombie, N., Hill, S., & Turner, B. S. (1984). *Dictionary of sociology* (2nd ed.) New York: Penguin.

Anderson, J. M. (1990). Health care across cultures. *Nursing Outlook*, *38*, 136–139.

Anthony-Tkach, C. (1981). Care of the Mexican-American patient. *Nursing & Health Care*, *2*, 424–427, 432.

Axtell, R. E. (1991). *Gestures: The do's and taboos of gestures and body language around the world.* New York: Wiley.

Bodner, A., & Leininger, M. (1992). Transcultural nursing care values, beliefs, and practices of American (USA) gypsies. *Journal of Transcultural Nursing*, *4*, 17–28.

Boyle, J. S., & Andrews, M. M. (1989). *Transcultural concepts in nursing care.* Glenview, IL: Scott, Foresman.

Bullough, V. L., & Bullough, B. (1982). *Health care for the other Americans.* New York: Appleton-Century-Crofts.

Carpio, B., & Majumdar, B. (1991). Putting culture into curricula. *The Canadian Nurse*, *8*, 32–33.

Davis, S. P. (1992). Africanity theory and the new student in nursing. *ABNF Journal*, *3*, 26–30.

DeSantis, L. (1991). Developing faculty expertise in culturally focused care and research. *Journal of Professional Nursing*, *7*, 300–309.

Galanti, G. (1991). *Caring for patients from different cultures: Case studies from American hospitals.* Philadelphia: University of Pennsylvania Press.

Giger, J. N., Davidhizar, R. E., & Turner, G. T. (1992). Black American folk medicine health care beliefs: Implications for nursing plans of care. *ABNF Journal*, *3*, 42–46.

Kluckhohn, F. R. (1976). Dominant and variant value orientations. In P. J. Brink (Ed.), *Transcultural nursing: A book of readings* (pp. 63–81). Englewood Cliffs, NJ: Prentice-Hall.

Leininger, M. M. (Ed.). (1991a). *Culture care diversity and universality: A theory of nursing.* New York: National League for Nursing Press.

Leininger, M. (1991b). Transcultural nursing: The study and practice field. *NSNA Imprint*, 55–66.

Platt, L. A., & Persico, Jr., V. R. (1992). *Grief in cross-cultural perspective: A casebook.* New York: Garland.

Rosenthal, M. M., & Frenkel, M. (1992). *Health care systems and their patients: An international perspective.* Boulder: Westview Press.

Ross-Gordon, J. M., Martin, L. G., & Briscoe, D. B. (Eds.). (1990). *Serving culturally diverse populations.* San Francisco: Jossey-Bass.

Saylor, C., & Taylor, T. (1993). Transformation nursing education and cultural diversity. *Nurse Educator*, *18*, 26–28.

Spector, R. E. (1991). *Cultural diversity in health and illness* (3rd ed.). Norwalk, CT: Appleton & Lange.

U.S. Commission on Civil Rights. (1970). *Racism in America and how to combat it.* Washington, DC: U.S. Government Printing Office.

U.S. Department of Commerce. Bureau of the Census. (1991). *Statistical abstract of the United States* (111th ed.). Washington, DC: U.S. Government Printing Office.

Weidman, H. H. (1979). The transcultural view: Prerequisite to interethnic (intercultural) communication in medicine. *Social Science and Medicine, 13B,* 85–87.

14

Health Care on
the Mexican–American Border

Patricia T. Castiglia

The United States has been making political and economic efforts to stimulate commerce with both its border neighbors, Canada and Mexico. The border area separating the U.S. and Mexico has many problems exacerbated by the clash between a high technology and a Third World country.

Issues related to health care along the U.S.–Mexico border have accelerated in terms of importance for the United States. One issue relates to the new North American Free Trade Agreement (NAFTA). This agreement will eliminate tariffs and other trade barriers between the United States, Mexico, and Canada. It will create a free trade zone of more than 360 million consumers. This agreement will have an impact not only on the transportation and communication infrastructures, but also on the health care infrastructure. The appeal of high-quality health care on the United States side of the border already exists. Even more women may decide to have their children born in the United States for the entitlements here. It is also anticipated that people from the interior of Mexico will move to border areas to take advantage of job opportunities. This migration may lessen, however, if more U.S. companies establish their businesses in the interior of Mexico.

Another issue which is predominant along this border relates to health care reform proposals. Will proposed programs cover undocumented workers already living in the United States? There are at least 5 million undocumented workers here at present. Statewide costs for undocumented California immigrants topped $700 million in 1992 and are expected to top $1 billion when the border becomes more open. The estimated health care, housing, energy assistance, education, welfare, and prison expenses for undocumented immigrants cost the United States

$5.4 billion dollars in 1990 (Geyer, 1993). Obviously, the greatest impact has occurred in border areas. When people appear with health problems requiring immediate care, ascertaining citizenship does not appear to be a major consideration.

What happens in health care along the U.S.-Mexico border and responsibility for administering health care to residents of the border are issues that will persist into the 21st century.

BORDER CHARACTERISTICS

People living along the U.S.–Mexico border are exposed on a daily basis to the threat of disease, environmental stress, and the lack of adequate economic resources to meet those needs. The border area is one of international transport, an area where the warm climate attracts many "sunbirds" from northern cities, and as a desert, an area with a fragile ecological balance.

The 2,000-mile border extends through four U.S. states—California, Arizona, New Mexico, and Texas—and through six Mexican states: Baja California; Sonora; Chihuahua; Coahuila; Monterrey; and Tamaulipas. The border stretches from the Pacific Ocean to the Gulf of Mexico and is one of the longest unfortified borders in the world (see Figure 14.1). The Rio Grande River (called the Rio Bravo in Mexico) serves as the border line for Texas and Mexico but it is scarcely a challenge to cross.

At the turn of the century there were an estimated less than100 thousand people living along the border. Today that population is about 10 million. Much of the area consists of desert terrain surrounded by "papier maché-like" mountains, that is, bare and brown with little vegetation and a "wrinkled" appearance. It is an environment where water resources are limited, where air pollution exists, and where there is no real boundary for water pollution, air pollution, or disease.

Many of the inhabitants are descendants of early frontiersmen. They are of Spanish, Mexican, and Anglo descent; often, they are of mixed heritage. Because of the pleasant, warm climate, the area is attractive to "snowbirds" escaping the severe northern winters, as well as to retirees seeking a warm climate and a relatively economical living style. Metropolitan areas are really transborder, and include El Paso, Texas and Juarez, Mexico with a population well over 1½ million; Laredo, Texas and Nuevo Laredo, Mexico with over 400,000 people; San Diego, California and Tijuana, Mexico with approximately 2 million people; and Imperial County, California and Mexicali, Mexico with over 600,000 people. The Mexican side of the border is one of the more prosperous areas of Mexico, while the American side consists of some of the poorest areas in the United States.

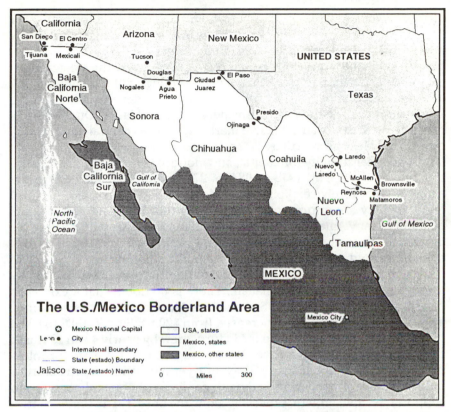

FIGURE 14.1 Map of the U.S.–Mexican border area.

ECONOMIC CONSIDERATIONS OF THE BORDER AREA

Trade, government, and services are the major industries along the border. Farming remains an important activity, with cotton the major crop in many areas. The falling peso in Mexico reduced wages, lowered production costs, and lured foreign industry. The income for border residents remains very low. For example, in 1986, the per capita income for Texas was $13,486 while it was $8,422 for Texas border residents (Shikles, 1988).

Representatives of both countries have been involved in working on the North American Free Trade Agreement (NAFTA). This effort was preceded in the 1960s by an international subcontracting industry (in-hand assembly). This became known as the *maquila* industry, a twin plant concept in which production components are carried out on both sides of the border. American-owned plants benefit from the large number of girls and women workers, many of whom have migrated to the border from the interior in search of work. They are hired because most of the assembly work in Mexico requires nimble fingers. After oil, the *maquilas* have become the largest source of foreign exchange for the Mexican government. They employ more than 475,000 young adults (Promoting binational cooperation, 1991). The key factor in the development of these industries has been the need for a cheap supply of labor. On the American side there exists an extensive market as well as capital and technology. On the Mexican side there is "socialized, trained and relatively cheap labor, political stability for capital, and modern facilities for administration and management" (Alba, 1984, p. 27). Some Mexicans believe the *maquilas* to be foreign exploitation of Mexico's poor economy. They also feel that they are unprotected as they venture into the international economy. Many Americans on the other hand perceive that jobs are being stolen because some jobs have been transferred to Mexico by U.S. companies, and that the American economy is threatened.

The free trade discussions have had to confront the issues of competition, cooperation and nationalism. There is no doubt that Mexico has benefitted, as has the United States, since Mexico opened its economy. U.S. exports to Mexico have increased from $20.6 billion in 1988 to $33.3 billion in 1991. Mexico's economy, in turn, grew by nearly 4% in 1991 and the stock market soared by over 100% (Padgett, 1992). A major problem persists for Mexico because it does not yet have the infrastructure—housing, roads, transportation, health care, environmental control—to support this rapid growth, especially along the border. The United States, while encouraging free trade, has not allocated economic resources to support the increased commerce. The American border states feel this should be a federal concern, as free trade is a national policy, and thus far, the federal government has not committed resources.

These economic policies have a direct bearing on the health status of people living along the border. Whether or not environmental problems and the health status of the residents can improve is tied to these issues.

ENVIRONMENTAL CONCERNS HAVING AN IMPACT ON HEALTH

It is obvious that an escalating population and economic growth are the major factors affecting people living along the border. These factors place demands upon the environmental resources of the land, ground water and surface water, and the quality of the air. All of these are affected by national, state, and international regulations.

At present, the entire surface flow of water for the border is fully appropriated, although the border population is expected to double by the year 2000 (Utton, 1984). Because the Rio Grande is a boundary, the border region is also governed by the International Boundary and Water Commission. Farming activities along the Rio Grande have had to be reduced due to new populations and economic growth, which in turn produces an escalating demand on surface water resources. Both sides of the border, especially in the El Paso-Juarez area, are pumping from groundwater reservoirs (aquifers) faster than they can be re-charged. Aquifers are being recharged at as little as 5% of the withdrawal. To protect this precious supply of ground water, regulation of land use must occur. Such regulation must be concerned not only with the quantity, but also the quality, of water, since the pollution of ground water has been traced to hazardous waste disposal.

It is important to note that the dangers from hazardous waste disposal are not confined to the border area alone. It is feared that sewage contamination may be spread throughout the United States markets through food supplies which have passed through border packing houses. These packing houses ship produce and seafood chilled with ice that may be contaminated by parasites and viruses (Solis & Nazario, 1992). Water treatment plants along the border are only capable of treating approximately 16% of the municipal and industrial waste water. Some cities, including Juarez the fifth largest city in Mexico, have no sewage system at all. It has been reported that 12 million gallons of raw sewage flows into the Tijuana River which then flows into the United States from Mexico. The City of Tijuana, Mexico has no water pollution problem, but well water in San Diego County, California has become increasingly contaminated (Warner, 1991).

Air pollution from unpaved roads, emissions from cars, due largely to the lack of emission controls in Mexico, from the burning of tires, wood and other materials in Mexico; and from uncontrolled industries continue to pollute the air. Much has been accomplished in controlling discharges from a smelter plant in El Paso, but much more needs to be done to raise the quality of air in El Paso to meet the U.S. Environmental Protection Agency's standards. When air inversions occur, a mantle hovers over the El Paso-Juarez area which is situated in a valley between the Sierra Madre and the Franklin Mountains.

The increased population migration to the border has stimulated the expansion of *colonias* on both sides of the border. *Colonias* are sprawling communities where, on the American side, people strive to achieve the American dream; that is, they try to acquire a piece of land and to build a home where their families can have a better life. They are usually American citizens of Mexican descent who have had a poor education and who work at very low-paying jobs. They construct the best homes they can, usually shacks. The lands they purchase with long-term leases have no water, no sewage disposal, unpaved roads and often no electricity. In addition, there is no transportation. Until recently land owners had contracts which allowed them to reclaim the land if even one monthly payment was missed.

Vector control is a problem for many areas along the border. When it rains or when water is released from the Rio Grande, ponds form, which are breeding places for mosquitos. In Juarez an 18-mile open sewage ditch 250 yards from the border has become one of the largest single mosquito sources in North America. Called Agua Negra, and the pond is sprayed daily by the El Paso City County Health Department, because, unfortunately, the mosquitos do not know to stay on their side of the Rio Grande (Nickey, 1989).

HEALTH PROBLEMS ALONG THE U.S.-MEXICO BORDER

Given the economic and environmental factors discussed above, it is easy to identify actual and potential health problems for border residents. The first problem, and the one that influences all aspects of health promotion, is the lack of access to good quality medical care on both sides of the border. For example, there is only one public hospital located on the 1000-mile border of Texas: R.E. Thomason General Hospital in El Paso. The next closest hospital is 250 miles away. Less than half the people along the border have private medical insurance and two thirds of the poor are not eligible for Medicaid (Promoting binational cooperation, 1991). Service for the elderly, adolescents, and those with mental health problems are especially limited.

Communicable diseases are persistent enemies. For example, tuberculosis rates in El Paso are twice the United States national average. Drug-resistant tuberculosis is a major problem on the Mexican side of the border. Syphilis also has a high incidence, but there are few cases of AIDS or gonorrhea. Because stray dogs are common on the Mexican side of the border, canine rabies is very prevalent, since the dogs, like the mosquitos, do not recognize the border. What helps to control rabies on the U.S. side is the major highway which parallels the Rio Grande River. Dogs are seldom successful in crossing this barrier alive.

Hepatitis A rates in Juarez approximate 100% by the time adulthood is reached. In a U.S. rural area east of El Paso, Hepatitis A has been found in 50% of children entering school and 100% of adults. Various forms of dysentery and intestinal parasites linked to poor sanitation are also prevalent. Preventable diseases, such as measles, continue to cause early death or disabilities in border children. Currently cholera is anticipated as it wends its way from Central America through Mexico, to the border. Its spread is inevitable given the lack of environmental controls. Cholera claimed approximately 4,000 lives in Latin American countries in 1991-92 and at least one case was confirmed in Brownsville, Texas (Kennedy, 1992).

Common health problems for Mexican American and Mexican women include obesity, diabetes, anemia, high blood pressure, and cervical cancer. The rate of cervical cancer in women in South Texas is the same high rate as that in for Latin America. A survey of Hispanic women in El Paso in 1991 found that 18% of the total number of women sampled (549) had never had a Pap smear and 65 percent had never had a mammogram (Mapula & Vasquez, 1991). In the United States breast cancer metastasis is reported to be at 50% but at R. E. Thomason General Hospital in El Paso, 73% of the women admitted for cancer have metastasis from breast cancer (Brown, 1989).

Forty-eight percent of people living along the border in 1985 were under 25 years old. This may be attributed to the influx of young immigrants from Mexico and other Central American countries, the high birth rate, and the relatively low infant death rate (Shikles 1988). There is a high fertility rate along the border although the rate has declined in the last two years and has declined in Mexico since the passage of the General Population Law of 1974 which allows birth control measures. Government programs, increased access to contraceptives, and private programs have all contributed to the decline in fertility rates. Despite this, the fertility rate of the 15 border counties is 93.7 per thousand women of child rearing age. This compares to 74.5 per thousand in the state of Texas. Almost 43% of these women have no prenatal care (Nickey, 1989).

Another factor influencing the low mortality rates for young Hispanics is the fact that few Mexican-American newborns are classified as low birth-weight. Infant mortalities have been at or below the national rates for people on this side of the border. Survival after birth is difficult, however, due to all the factors related to poverty—malnutrition, unsanitary living conditions, and a lack of medical care, especially preventive care (see Table 14.1). Recently newborn anencephaly has become a cause of alarm in Brownsville, Texas. In the Spring of 1991, three anencephalic babies were born in a 36-hour period. The Centers for Disease Control report that this condition usually occurs at a rate of 10.4 per 10,000 (Geyer, 1993). In comparison the Brownsville area has had rates of 16.66 per 10,000 in 1989; 30.16 per 10,000 in 1990; and 11.59 per 10,000 in 1991 (Researchers fear Mexican air, 1992). Most of the mothers of these infants reportedly lived within a 2.4-mile radius of the Rio Grande River. Matamoros, Mexico is the sister city of Brownsville, and the factories there discharge xylene, toluene, and other pollutants into the air. These

TABLE 14.1 Mortality Rates per 100,000 Persons*

Population	AGES			
	1–14	15–44	45–64	65–
United States (all races)	33.8	137.3	893.3	5,153.3
Border area (all races)	30.6	119.0	705.4	4,094.7
White border	42.3	147.9	873.3	4,282.0
Hispanic border	27.9	109.5	606.6	3,901.9

*Adapted from: Shikles, J. L. (1988). Texas Border Area Health Care. Report to Senator Lloyd Bentsen, Washington, DC: United States General Accounting Office, October, 26, 1988, p. 22.

substances are common in electronics plants and are also by-products of gasoline refining.

A number of Mexican women choose to have their children on the U.S. side of the border. Although many of them do so to bestow U.S. citizenship, others do so because they feel the natal and postnatal care is better here. Because many mothers and babies return to Mexico, it is impossible to acquire accurate mortality rates. One of the problems along the border is the virtually unregulated practice of lay midwives. In El Paso County alone, lay midwives deliver approximately 1,500 women each year. In an 18- month study there were 31 complications in these deliveries. Of these, nine babies, not counting deaths or status epilepticus babies, cost taxpayers approximately $1 million each (Brown, 1989).

Problems of the adolescent years have become of great concern along the border. Violence and gang-related crimes are increasing. Teenage pregnancy, alcohol use, and other substance abuse problems are common. Young people with no money, no jobs, and no transportation often have no hope for a future. Gangs provide them with an identity, a sense of belonging, and reinforce the adolescent belief in indestructibility. Few Mexican-Americans use mental health resources, and few studies have been done on mental health problems of Mexican-Americans. A study by Canales and Roberts (1987) suggests that Mexican-Americans exhibit substantial symptoms of depression and anxiety.

The *maquilas* have the opportunity to improve the health of female employees. However, reports of excessive noise levels, exposure to toxic chemicals, poor ventilation, and few rest periods have been made (Promoting binational cooperation, 1991). Some *maquilas* provide health care and education for their employees and their families; many often include all persons living in the area of the plant for immunizations. Federal programs such as the Special Supplemental Food Program for Women, Infants, and Children (WIC), the Maternal and Infant Health Improvement Act for high risk mothers and infants, family planning services, and other federal and state programs help residents, but are subject to budget cuts. These services also are suspect for non resident aliens who fear deportation.

HEALTH CARE IN MEXICO

Mexico does have a national health care system, but access problems persist. Mexicans who have high incomes obviously can seek and obtain the best that private care has to offer, both in Mexico and in the United States. Middle-class people, those having government jobs, employees of large firms, and residents of certain communal agricultural communities, have access to the Instituto Mexicano de Seguro Social, Social Security, or, if government employees, to the Instituto de Seguridad y Servicios Sociales Para los Trabajadores del Estado clinics and hospitals. These two sources of care provide for less than half the population of the Mexican border.

The remainder of the population, 50–60%, is covered by the Servicios Coordinado de Salud Publico en los Estados, the Health and Welfare Ministry. Care in these clinics might be given by physicians or nurses filling the required year of service after completing their education. This is called the *pasante* year. In more rural areas, nurses or *promotoras* are the usual care givers. Hospitals for the poor are not usually well-staffed and often lack more advanced technology.

All movement for health care is not from Mexico to the United States. Some physicians in the U.S. send their patients to Mexico to save them money. In Mexico, for example, ultrasound costs $20 as compared to $150 in the United States. Via PROFAX, a binational program located in Brownsville, Americans can obtain vasectomies or tubal ligations in Mexico for a cost of $3.00 to $5.00. A number of Americans also go to Mexico for dental care, dentures, and to obtain medications. Many medications (e.g., penicillin) do not require prescriptions in Mexico, and drugs usually cost much less.

EFFORTS TO IMPROVE BORDER HEALTH

The Environmental Protection Agency (EPA) and the Mexican environmental agency, the Secretary of Urban Development and Ecology (SEDUE), are collaborating on a plan to preserve environmental quality on the border. It is called the U.S.-Mexico Integrated Environmental Plan.

Both agencies involved in the plan, however, have limited budgets. The pollution control budget for the entire country of Mexico is $3.15 million— less than the pollution budget for the state of Texas (Smith, 1991).

As a beginning effort to develop the plan, a series of hearings were conducted on both sides of the border by EPA and SEDUE. It is obvious to everyone that the increased population and economic growth along the border will continue to strain the infrastructure. Control measures needed include: water and waste water treatment plants, pollution control equipment, hazardous waste disposal, and the conservation of all resources (Smith, 1991). Mexico's law on Ecological Equilibrium and Environmental Protection requires that any company wishing to operate in Mexico must submit an environmental impact statement and risk analysis. In addition, Mexico will not allow businesses which have been rejected by other nations because of dangers to the environment to operate in Mexico (Smith, 1991).

Environmental and public health issues are also addressed by the U.S.- Mexico Border Health Association and a number of privately funded projects. The U.S.-Mexico Border Health Association attempts to coordinate policies on public health activities and to improve communication between local health departments from both sides of the border. EPA and SEDUE are mandated to cooperate in efforts by the August 1983 La Paz agreement. Both national governments have delegated mediation of boundary and water conflicts along the border to the International Boundary and Water Commission, founded in 1889.

Many people involved with public health and environmental issues along the border believe that there should be a permanent U.S–Mexico Border Health and Environmental Commission. A great deal of private, charitable care for border residents is given by educational and health service organizations. Private foundations such as the Kellogg, Ford, Robert Wood Johnson, Kaiser, Pew Memorial Trust, and the Hogg Foundation, have invested considerable resources to improve conditions along the border. These efforts have thus far been able to make only a dent in the great need for services. Both governments must invest resources if the border health problems are to be curtailed. Suggestions such as development and user fees on foreign assembly plants may be resources to finance the needed infrastructure development.

The majority of the border area counties have shortages of physicians, dentists, nurses, and all other health care providers. Efforts are being made to develop new models of health care to better provide for the needs of border residents through the Community Partnership project of the W. K. Kellogg Foundation. In this project, young people living along the border will be assisted in pursuing preparation as health care professionals and will hopefully practice in these areas.

NURSING'S ROLE IN BORDER HEALTH

The U.S.–Mexico border residents have long been invisible at both the federal and state health planning levels. Many of the residents have such limited access to health care that it is difficult to believe that they are residents of an advanced nation such as the United States. It is important to consider health needs along the border, as it is clearly not a local problem, but rather a national concern.

The role for professional nurses involved in health care along the U.S.-Mexico border is challenging. Health promotion and disease prevention activities, such as health fairs, where screening procedures are available, and immunization clinics, are important components of a comprehensive approach to health care. Primary care must be provided in areas where the people live, for example, in schools, churches, and empty stores. The lack of transportation and the limited financial resources means that most of the residents of the border seek episodic care at the emergency room of the city/county hospital. Many conditions could be prevented or minimized if primary care services were available. Follow-up care for those seen in the emergency room is almost non existent.

Nurses must be advocates for the many disenfranchised people living along the U.S.-Mexico border. They must be informed about health care policy legislation and must participate in activities to promote the improved health status of border residents. The scope of the nurse's role has broadened to include public issues related to the health and welfare of all people. Nurses must be creative in developing strategies for providing holistic health care. In addition to having a strong knowledge base and excellent clinical skills, they must also develop cultural sensitivity.

SUMMARY

The U.S.–Mexico border is an example of collision of two worlds two nations, two cultures, two economies, and two political structures. Commingling of problems and benefits occur. Health and environmental problems are serious. There is no way to prevent, nor is there a desire to prevent, commerce across a border that is little more than a delineation on a map. El Paso alone has over 40 million legal, one-way, border crossings per year from Mexico to the U.S. each year. Many workers return to Mexico at the end of the work day, and a large number of illegal entries to the U.S. occur daily.

If the United States is to be truly international, if the welfare of all U.S. citizens is important, then the problems related to health and environment along the border must be solved. Economic growth depends on this resolution; concern for human rights demands it.

TOPICS FOR DISCUSSION

1. At the present time, tax laws and other incentives encourage American companies moving across the Mexican border or establishing *maquila* industries which parallel the border. What is your opinion on this matter?
2. The busy border facilitates the spread of epidemics from one side to the other. What diseases would you anticipate might cross the border? Why?
3. Describe the water problems of the border area. What factors make water such a problem?
4. What are some of the cultural differences between Mexicans and Americans that might have an impact on health or health care?

REFERENCES

Alba, F. (1984) Mexico's Northern border: A framework of reference. In C. Sepulveda and A. E. Utton (Eds.), *U.S.-Mexico Border Region: Anticipating Resource Needs and Issues to the Year 2000* (pp. 31–35). El Paso, TX: Texas Western Press and The Center for Inter-American and Border Studies.

Brown, J. (1989). The border: Where public health meets primary care. In Border Health Conference Proceedings, El Paso, TX: Texas Medical Association.

Canales, G., & Roberts, R. E. (1987). Gender and mental health in the Mexican origin population of South Texas: Mental health issues of the Mexican origin population in Texas. Proceedings of The Fifth Robert Lee Sutherland Seminar in Mental Health (pp. 89–99). Austin, TX: University of Texas.

Geyer, G. A. (1993, May 9). Do we really want to pay huge health tabs for non-U.S. citizens? *El Paso Times*, p. 2G.

Kennedy, J. M. (1992, July 6). Health care crisis worsening along border. *Austin American Statesman*, pp. A1, A13.

Mapula, C., & Vasquez, C. (1991). Preliminary results from community cancer survey among Hispanic women in El Paso, 1991. Unpublished analysis conducted by the Texas Department of Health.

Nickey, L. N. (1989). *Welcome.* Texas Medical Association—Border Health conference, August 23–24, 1989. El Paso, TX, Border Health Conference Proceedings.

Padgett, T. (1992, March 23). The gloom behind the boom. *Newsweek*, p. 48.

Promoting binational cooperation to improve health along the U.S.-Mexico border. (1991). *Carnegie Quarterly.* 26,1–16.

Researchers fear Mexican air causes Brownsville birth defects. (1992, May 3). *El Paso Times*, p. A1.

Shikles, J. L. (1988) *Texas border area health care: Report to Senator Lloyd Bentsen.* Washington, DC: United States General Accounting Office, October 26, 1988, 1-53.

Smith, R. B. (1991) Mexico: Challenge and opportunity. *Occupational Health & Safety, 60,* 42-44.

Solis, D., & Nazario, S. L. (1992, Febuary 25). U.S., Mexico take on border pollution. *Wall Street Journal,* pp. B1, B8.

Utton, A. C. (1984). *Overview.* In C. Sepulveda and A. E. Utton (Eds.), *U.S.-Mexico border region*: Anticipating resource needs and issues to the year 2000 (pp. 7–19). El Paso, TX: Texas Western Press and the Center for Inter-American and Border Studies.

Warner, D. C. (1991). Health issues at the U.S.–Mexican border. *Journal of the American Medical Association, 265,* 242–247.

15

Conveying Professionalism: Working Against the Old Stereotypes

Nancy Campbell-Heider, Cynthia Allen Hart, and Martha Dewey Bergren

Language and dress in all organizations emerge as metaphors of the existing work culture and provide symbolic cues about individuals that can enhance or refute social power. Prior to the 19th century, nurses belonged primarily to religious groups and as such adopted the robes of their orders to symbolize their status. Similarly, 19th-century women used formal social address as a mechanism to communicate the image of the "traditional lady" of the era. The status of "lady" implied power denied to other women and allowed early nurses who adopted this image to demand respect from men (Bullough, 1990).

As nursing evolved into a separate discipline with primarily nonreligious ties, early "nurses" needed a mechanism to set themselves apart from the masses of untrained and often illiterate caregivers. To accomplish this task, Nightingale, who never wore a uniform herself, instituted dress codes for her students to distinguish the new trained nurse from the untrained camp followers. Emerging nursing schools in the United States also adopted the Nightingale model and the white dress, cap, stockings, and shoes soon became the professional standard (Blumhagen, 1979; Kalisch & Kalisch, 1985).

Today's nurses rightfully have more control over their apparel and the level of formality in their bedside communications. Modern nurses are wearing less traditional clothing and using more informal communications with patients than their predecessors. Most apparent in the nurse—patient realm is the current tendency for nurses to be on a first-name basis with their patients and to adopt less traditional uniforms or street clothing. This chapter suggests that nurses' verbal informality with patients is linked to persistent stereotypic themes that diminish the professional image, shroud the cognitive nature of their work, perpetuate hierarchical relationships between physicians and nurses, and even threaten nurses' therapeutic effectiveness. Conversely, the shedding of the formal nurse uniform may have some opposite effects.

Professional characteristics in any discipline include the following factors: a social mandate for the discipline; a professional society that maintains control over the standards of practice; a defined scope of practice and body of specialized knowledge; the ability to control entry into the discipline; and group members' acceptance of a common ideology or societal mission (Baszanger, 1985). Schutzenhofer (1988) notes that the attainment of autonomy has been difficult for nurses who, by virtue of their identity as a traditionally female discipline, embody feminine characteristics that are inconsistent with traditional images of professionalism. For some, the integration of professional roles produces conflict with traditional female socialization. Women are not expected to display masculine characteristics of ambition, achievement, competitiveness, or autonomy (Rosenow, 1988). This situation is not compatible with professional socialization; however, it may explain some of the reluctance of women to assert themselves socially in the professional world. By playing down social status, a nurse professional can remain feminine while participating in a professional role.

Styles (1982) distinguishes between the attainment of a collective professionalism and individual professionhood. Professionalism embodies the collective character of a group, whereas professionhood focuses on the characteristics of the individual and suggests that "professionalism of nursing will be achieved only through the professionhood of its members" (p.8). This theory implies the need for emphasis on the personal presentation of every nurse in every type of practice, as it is the individual nurse who fosters our collective image. And this issue reinforces the importance of verbal and nonverbal symbolism related to *naming* and *clothing*.

STEREOTYPING PROFESSIONAL ROLES

The process of stereotyping professional roles results from complex interactions related to social cognition theories that involve the development of "schema" or mental pictures to interpret work roles (Kaler, Levy, & Schall,1989). Societal stereotypes bias the processing and interpretation of this information, which implies that altering the image of nurses must include the development of new, and more positive, nurse schemata. Research and public opinion polls regarding societal views of nurses indicate that the public still views nurses as nuturant (feminine) and concerned for others, but only moderately well educated. Physicians, by contrast, are characterized by both high achievement (masculine) and high educational attainment (Kaler et al., 1989). A helping orientation should be a desirable stereotype to reinforce, as many nurses argue that this caring dimension is the essence of nursing. However, this quality apparently overshadows nurses' images as intelligent and autonomous professionals.

Feminist authors Gordon and Buresh (1991) question whether nurses can reach equality with physicians when the public and press view caring as women's work and nurses as physicians' handmaidens. They report that Americans perceive the health care system as primarily biomedical phenomena. Physicians conquer disease and nurses are nice and caring. The press has trouble finding words to describe the cognitive nature of nursing, as caring techniques appear less exciting than curing roles. Most people fail to recognize that major medical conditions such as AIDS, Alzheimer's disease, and other chronic illnesses represent significant nursing problems. Bullough's (1992) analysis of the trends in nursing specialty practices describes the branching of advanced practitioners—nurse practitioners, nurse-midwives, nurse anesthetists, and critical care nurses—into those who treat and those—clinical specialists—who provide more traditional types of care. This division in nurse ideology may herald a new era that allows the general public to view nurses as practitioners who care for and treat many types of conditions previously in the exclusive purview of the physician. A strong presentation of professionalism when coupled with this expert clinical care is a promising beginning for educating society about the true value of nursing.

THE MEANING OF LANGUAGE
IN SOCIETY AND THE WORKPLACE

There is considerable emphasis in contemporary writing about the importance of language, particularly as it relates to reinforcing sex-role stereotypes (Sampselle, 1990). Social interaction is the most common source of social control, especially in relation to nonverbal and subtle environmental cues (Henley & Freeman, 1988) and nonverbal communication is four times more powerful than verbal interaction when it comes to influencing a social exchange. Women are particularly sensitive to this form of communication. When sexist themes manifest in the hospital realm, nurses are frequently depicted as relational to the physician and their professional stature is converted into the well-known "handmaiden" image. Nurses reinforce this image when they use their first names with patients, whereas physicians retain their professional titles. Physicians known as "Doctor" and nurses as "Mary" provide verbal imaging of the social distance and hierarchical relations between the two disciplines.

The complexity of addressing nurses in the hospital setting is humorously and pointedly described by Vincenzi (1991) in an assumed role of "Nurse Manners." She recommends that nurses at the bedside separate business etiquette from social conversation to avoid "instant intimacy." When nurses introduce themselves to patients by their first names, they are socially relegated to a position of deference, not unlike that of servants who are usually addressed by their first names. This communication message is particularly poignant in the presence of other professionals who retain their "Dr." or "Ms." status and sets the stage for hierarchical power relationships between patients, physicians, and nurses. Figure 15.1 illustrates how nurses assume subordinate social status when their titles are not parallel with physicians and patients. This problem is compounded when physicians address nurses by their first names and nurses respond with the professional title of doctor (Henly & Freeman, 1988). The nurse's loss of personal power is often experienced unconsciously, and can encourage submissiveness to physicians and confusion in patients, who are unprepared for social intimacy in therapeutic relationships (Figure 15.1).

Since society continues to devalue the work of women and traditional female roles, many nurses unconsciously accept this situation and think of themselves as "just a nurse" or just "Mary." The once professional appellation of Miss, Mrs., or Nurse Smith, which now might include Ms., Mr. , Nurse, or Dr. Smith, is replaced by first names or even worse, nicknames. This response is consistent with the literature documenting the strategies that subordinate groups typically employ to cope with their second-class status in organizations and society (Hedin, 1986; Miller & Mothner, 1976; Roberts, 1983). It is interesting to note that in the popular science fiction realm of *Star Trek: The Next Generation*, the old fashioned title of *Nurse* is used to provide this crew member equal status with all others on the *Enterprise*. Apparently *nurse doctors* are not *yet* the norm in the 24th century!

SYMBOLS OF SOCIAL DOMINANCE

Among nurses, oppressed group behavior manifests in negative themes that denigrate nurses and glorify dominant groups. Horizontal violence—or the tendency for subordinate groups to direct their frustration toward co-workers rather than dominant forces—might account for the reluctance of some nurses to recognize the status of those nurses who do obtain advanced educational degrees and other symbols of achievement,

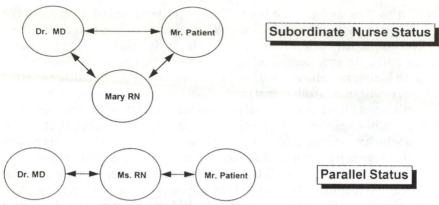

FIGURE 15.1. Communicating social status.

such as membership in honor societies and certification, in their intro-
ductions and written communications. Nurses are beginning to recognize
the benefit to the entire nursing profession of "advertising" that nurses
are also clinical specialists, certified, and doctorally prepared. However,
some reinforce the commonalties of nurses, rather than promoting individual accomplishments. Undervaluing of nurses by nurses lowers self-
esteem and can account for the tendency of many nurses to downplay
their association with their profession (Fagin & Diers, 1983).

Public evidence of low self-esteem among nurses discourages young
people from selecting this profession as it is assumed that nurses are
neither financially rewarded nor appropriately respected. This problem
was addressed on a national level by the ANA in a media campaign that
focused public attention on the essential nature and complexity of nursing care, as well as the benefits and rewards inherent in this career.
Nurses at the bedside must support these media messages by behavior
that conveys strong professional orientation.

NURSE–PATIENT INTERACTIONS

Benner and Wrubel (1989) developed their primacy of caring theory of
nursing to highlight the value of scientific knowledge and clinical judg-
ments that go unnoticed in most acute care areas that focus solely on
dramatic physician procedures. They discuss the necessity of "presencing"
with patients and families to foster patient understanding and support,
while allowing the patient to view nurses as knowledgeable workers
who are responsible for providing a safe and enabling environment. The
language used with patients must be one of "commitment, meanings,

skills, concerns and aspirations" (p.398). This type of meaningful language is very different from social language, such as the use of informal "chit-chat" involving the nurses' life. These types of conversations can lead to a loss of nurse objectivity and overinvolvement with patients, which interferes with care.

Peplau's (1952) now classic work on nurse–patient interactions emphasizes the intimate nature of nursing situations. In this context, the symbols of language—verbal and nonverbal—become especially significant metaphors of the hospital culture. When nurses use their first names, they often address patients by first names. Patients sometimes encourage use of their first names to reestablish parallel communications. This situation leads to a loss of individual identities that can redefine the therapeutic relationship into one with a more social emphasis. Using a diminutive of false familiarity also can exaggerate the existing gap that currently exists between the physically well and knowledgeable caregiver and the disabled and dependent patient (Zola, 1987).

Some nurses believe that using their last names increases personal vulnerability, which is understandable in today's violent society that still "allows" exploitation of females. Nurses should not need to mask their self-identity in the workplace in order to feel protected. This situation raises many questions about the social progress of modern women vis-à-vis institutional and societal violence against women. The denial of self-identity to insure safety could be viewed as a modern female strategy to cope with workplace vulnerability, which also manifests interpersonal control of women workers' social status. It would be particularly interesting to examine this theory in light of our historical use of formality in language and dress to protect nurses from harassment mentioned earlier in this chapter. If self-protection is the rationale behind first names for female nurses, this situation has many implications for therapeutic communications, but does not explain why female physicians, schoolteachers, and other professional women do not use the same strategies. Also, self-protection theories would not explain the prevalence of first-name use in male nurses.

NURSE–PHYSICIAN INTERACTIONS

The control of status titles in medicine has a long and interesting history. Physicians in the 18th century in Europe recognized that the title "doctor" was accorded those teachers who attained the highest academic degrees. Consequently, aspiring physicians adopted this title as a deliberate strategy designed to advance their professional status. Physicians are now so dominant in society that others who attain academic doctorates—particularly in the hospital setting—are sometimes intimidated about referring to themselves as doctors. These status discrepancies are frequently reinforced by organizational cultures in clinical settings that reinforce physicians' titling prerogatives, but overlook the social status credentials of others. The rationale for this behavior is nebulous, but it appears that some physicians "worry" that patients might confuse a nonphysician doctor with a physician. Apparently, this concern prompted organized medicine in Massachusetts to attempt to push through regulations that would mandate nonphysician providers to wear a badge specifying that they were not doctors, that is, medical doctors, and to list the name of their supervising physician (Reverby, 1987). It is unclear how this regulation would benefit consumers, as it is already standard practice for nonphysician health providers to list their credentials on a name badge. The listing of a supervising physician is both demeaning and unnecessary for those practitioners who are independently licensed.

Some nurses contend that social formalities are not necessary and that verbal symbolism is unimportant when interacting with patients or other professionals. However, Campbell-Heider and Pollock (1987) assert that the nurse–physician relationship is already characterized by deeply rooted male–female socialization themes that do interfere with the collegial nature of relationships. Certainly, the verbal reinforcement of the nurse as less worthy of formal introduction serves in many situations to maintain this negative status quo.

The literature on nurse-physician teams stresses that collegiality is an essential dimension and that patient outcomes are greatly improved when there is shared decision-making and mutual respect for clinical abilities between physicians and nurses (Baggs & Ryan, 1990; Baggs & Schmitt, 1988). Symbolic of this mutuality is the maintenance of parallel status when talking with patients and among themselves. In other words, nurses should be addressed in the same manner as their physician counterparts. If formal titles are used for physicians, the same behaviors should be used to address nurses. Such symbolism reinforces the interdependence and collegial nature of the team and provides for mutual respect. This message to patients can help to abolish persistent negative stereotypes about nurses.

This thinking is also consistent with recent literature advocating an abolishment of the traditional "doctor–nurse" game that carefully maintains the status differentials between physicians and nurses (Stein, Watts, & Howell, 1990). Social changes including the 1) diminishing public esteem for physicians; 2) increasing numbers of women in medicine; 3) the glut of physicians in light of a shortage of nurses; 4) more powerful and positive TV media images of nurses in series such as *China Beach* ; 5) increased advanced education and certification into specialties among nurses; and 6) new case management roles for nurses are altering physician-nurse relationships. New depictions of the old game must provide nurses with equal social status, which will facilitate more collegiality in practice as well. The principal vehicle for change is advanced nurse education and socialization of nursing students to relate to physicians in an assertive and direct manner. Unfortunately, nurse assertiveness is sometimes diminished by other communication behaviors that continue to imply second-class status.

THE MEANING OF CLOTHING

Dress, like language, is also a symbol for age, class, status, education, role, and professional autonomy (Goffman, 1959). Historically, the white uniform facilitated the identification of the nurse, which promoted the professional image by separating the *trained* from the *untrained* practitioners. This situation was most apparent when there were only three types of healthcare workers in the hospital and three distinct "uniforms": male physicians in white coats; female nurses in white dresses and caps; and nonmedical staff in a variety of occupation-specific clothing. The present proliferation of types of health care professionals and ancillary workers who wear variations on the traditional white uniform now diminishes the uniform's power to communicate a professional identity. This situation, coupled with the growing number of male nurses and rapidly increasing cadre of female physicians, further complicates the traditional uniform standard. Several authors suggest that the stethoscope, not the uniform, is more linked to professional nurse status than any other clinical garb (Hardin & Benton, 1984; Little, 1984).

THE COSTS AND BENEFITS OF UNIFORMS

Sociologists who study perception and responses to clothing consider uniforms a unique category of attire that embody many social messages. All clothing, but especially uniforms, shape the first impression of an individual by providing cues that an observer can link to stereotypes. Uniforms are symbols of group identity and such dress codes can be either informal or formal in nature. Even within a specified group, special markings or colors on a formal uniform designate particular status. All uniforms are characterized by a few items that are considered as the most salient social symbols: for example, the policeman's badge, physician's stethoscope, nurse's cap, chef's hat, and the like. The fact that many groups adopt uniforms or particular characteristics of uniforms to present a nonverbal message, such as the Salvation Army's adaptation of military dress, demonstrates the social power of clothing (Kaiser, 1990).

The organizational image and values associated with a particular type of clothing often assume more significance than other practical concerns. Certainly, the nurse's cap demonstrates this phenomenon. Most modern nurses now agree that the cap is a historical symbol that lacks relevance in today's practice environment. Characteristics of clothing such as color, style, and association with the most powerful groups also provide social messages. In fact, clothing can be imbued with many interpersonal qualities; the female in a skirted suit is associated with more male characteristics, such as forcefulness and decisiveness, than is the woman in a dress (Forsythe, Drake, & Cox, 1984). This situation poses many problems for women entering many traditional work settings in which the business *uniform* of men is well established. To compensate, many women, particularly those new in a field, chose to adopt clothing with many salient male characteristics—such as a tailored jacket. As women become more comfortable, powerful, and skilled in a field, they are freer to use more traditionally female clothing.

The benefits of uniforms to identify members of a group also has a downside. The visual characteristics of dress that designate the occupational category are usually based on social schema (Davis, 1990) constructed from stereotypes that serve to reduce the complexity of roles and uncertainty in communications. Once people are identified with a stereotypic notion, their individuality tends to be diminished, and the group's characteristics attributed without qualification (Raven & Rubin, 1976). Furthermore, such stereotypes are resistant to contradictory information (Stephan, 1985). Additional information learned about the person is used to *reinforce* rather than *refute* existing notions. The traditional white uniform of the female nurse is a significant salient characteristic that can link modern nurses to past themes, which are not all consistent with professional imaging. Likewise, the widespread adoption of colored, flowered, or other more casual "uniforms" can also link nurses with traditionally nonprofessional workers.

Although nursing uniforms once provided clear symbols of professionalism, historians report that the traditional white uniform now symbolizes the portrayal of nurses as angels of mercy, and handmaidens or servants to the physician (Kalisch & Kalisch, 1987; Muff, 1988), which create expectations that nurses are submissive, self-sacrificing, and unquestioning. Patients who respond to salient characteristics of uniforms that signal traditional stereotypes don't expect nurses to possess professional characteristics. It is this type of preconceived notion that drives some patients to ask "Why are you *just* a nurse?" (Diers, 1992).

The public is also unprepared for the nurse to be male, as the same stereotypic images cannot be applied to men, making some patients more uncomfortable with the social uncertainty associated with male nurses' roles (Brookfield, Douglas, Shapiro, & Clas, 1982; Kearns, 1986). Therefore, the current view that uniforms project the professional image of the nurse is based on the premise that the traditional social stereotypes and cultural context of the early 1900s still prevail. In reality, the uniform projects the *stereotypic image* and not the reality of nurses as autonomous providers with a high level of education and scientific expertise.

The uniform is also indicative of external monitoring of professional behavior, which is inconsistent with the role of the autonomous professional (Joseph, 1986). The underlying message of the dress code is that nurses cannot be trusted (Martin, Martin, & Sangster, 1986). Many nurse administrators resort to strict dress codes because they are frustrated by the failure of some nurses to adopt appropriate clothing. However, problems with sloppy attire and lack of professional presencing are best solved through more effective professional socialization. Strategies to address such problems require an emphasis on peer influence, increased professional orientation during nursing education, increased nurse empowerment by management, and examination of professional imaging through scholarly discourse. Nurse managers must also recognize that removing dress codes will require a period of transition and that some nurses might initially fail to make appropriate choices. Certainly, clothing choices could be optimized by appropriate preparations for dress code changes. Focus groups and presentations that explore the professional dynamics of clothing and allow for small group interaction to discuss what types of street clothing might be introduced to various clinical areas offer one possible mechanism to facilitate elimination of uniforms.

Uniforms do symbolize that the individual belongs to a specific group and accepts the norms and roles inherent in that profession. However, this situation can also influence the wearer and encourage nurses to assume *expected* roles (Joseph, 1986). The 1980s emphasis on power dressing is eroding the prestige of all types of uniforms (Kalisch & Kalisch, 1985). And most professional groups do not adhere to prescribed dress. This situation tends to relegate only lower level workers to uniform codes, and might explain why some patients view their nurse as more of a servant than a healthcare provider.

The uniform can also downplay the need for the individual to demonstrate skills and competencies (Szasz, 1982). Sparrow (1991) found that modern nurses who preferred the uniform were more task-oriented and likely to accept medical domination than those who preferred street clothes. Nurses working in street clothing were oriented to interpersonal relations and tended to work a multidisciplinary partnership. Other studies suggest that nurses with the least experience have the strongest preference for uniforms (Siegal, 1968; Smoothy, Nightingale & Harries, 1989). Today, unlike in the past, the uniform seems more representative of nurses with the *least* experience and education. However, it is unclear whether uniformed nurses consciously select this practice, or if organizational cultures encourage it to reinforce entrenched beliefs about the nature of professional nursing and maintain the status quo in interdisciplinary relationships. If this notion is correct, the white uniform may be sending some mixed messages about nursing as an equal opportunity profession that could serve to discourage males and nontraditional females from entering nursing. Perhaps this situation explains why a greater proportion of male nurses are attracted to the specialties mental health, anesthesia, and administration where there is an absence of special clothing that signifies the nurse (Flanagan, 1982). When patients encounter nurses practicing in nontraditional garb or street clothes, their communications are not immediately marred by preconceived role relationships. Nurses are free to use other types of communications to indicate professional status.

PATIENT PREFERENCES

A recent study evaluated the preference for female nurse uniforms by patients, nurses, and hospital administrators in regard to images of competence, efficiency, caring, and professional reliability (Magnum, Garrison, Lind, Thackeray, & Wyatt, 1991). Subjects gave the highest image rating to the nurse wearing white pants, a stethoscope draped around her neck, and a traditional white nurse's cap. Traditional symbols once exclusively associated with male physicians (pants and stethoscope) and female nurses (cap) remain meaningful indicators of professional abilities. However, as Bergren (1992) argues, patients' preferences for uniforms is understandable, as the uniform conforms to preconceived and comfortable images and beliefs about nurse role and status.

Also relevant to patients' interpretations of nurse dress is the notion that clothing must be matched to *social reality* (Kaiser, 1990). This means that clothing must be appropriately symbolic; a dinner dress at the bedside is not functional for physical care, and patients would unconsciously recognize this as a manipulation. However, the theory that a uniform is more serviceable than all types of street clothes must also be examined, in light of the fact that many of today's fashions are as functional, washable, and hygienic as the traditional uniform. This literature review failed to find any studies that address this basic issue. However, the concept of developing germproof clothing is explored in a recent article in the *American Journal of Nursing*. Burlington's new Bioguard™ treats fabric with an ammonium antimicrobial that resists colonization with *Staph aureus, E. coli, Klebsiella pneumoniae*, and *pseudomonas aeruginosa*; however, there is little evidence that uniforms cause spread of infection. The majority of infection control literature focuses on the need for good handwashing and latex gloves as the major barriers to nosocomial disease ("safe uniform" debate, 1986).

When hygiene is critical, nurses and other providers use special clothing, such as scrub suits, and clothes are changed before leaving the hospital. This type of practice promotes hygiene and equality among workers, which might explain the tendency for nurses in such specialized units to have higher morale and self-images than in situations where nurse identity is more circumscribed by traditional uniforms. Most critics of the uniform conclude that the white uniform does not need to be completely abandoned if still functional (MacFarlane, 1990; Martin et al., 1986; Szasz, 1982); however, the meaning of traditional attire must be evaluated in light of other nonverbal nuances.

REDEFINING THE NURSING WORK ENVIRONMENT

The work environment usually supports systems that have horizontal and vertical status divisions which display these values by fashion, custom, decorum, politeness, and language (Goffman, 1959). In all types of nursing care settings, nurses' presentation of self allow others to predict knowledge, professional skills, general behaviors, and social status.

Barker (1991) calls for a nursing social architecture that develops self-esteem and professional values. This social architecture must provide an organizational identity, personal empowerment, and a common ideology about nursing professionalism. The development of a common ideology that promotes professional autonomy and maturity requires leaders who strive to activate nurses' abilities to display their professional competence and professionalism.

Some suggest that shaping the work cultures within large organizations are a prime management role (Peters & Waterman, 1982). Once the structure and technology of a unit is in place, the development of group ideology and language to support these beliefs should follow. Language and dress communicate the organization's beliefs about the nature and power of groups within an organization, and become metaphors of the underlying work culture of an institution. Environmental cues set the stage for interactions where status differentials are reinforced or refuted.

The recent nurse shortage highlights the social mandate for nursing services, but re-emphasizes the difficulties nurses still encounter in many work environments. Barker (1991) suggests that a new paradigm in nursing leadership is needed to transform the typically hierarchical hospital organizations into more engaging structures that will encourage the professional advancement and empowerment of nurses to occur. Her transformational strategies are based on a model developed by Bennis and Nanus (1985) and include four components: (1) creating a vision or collective purpose for the nursing department; (2) providing a "social architecture" that fosters collegial and participatory relationships among workers; (3) creating an atmosphere of organizational trust; and most importantly, 4) developing a cadre of leaders and staff with high self-esteem and the capabilities to empower others.

The decision by nurses to use informal titling with patients and clinical attire that depicts outdated professional images are symptomatic of cultural learning that decreases self-esteem among practicing nurses. Bedside manner is the product of female, professional, and organizational socialization. Figure 15.2 depicts these relationships; however, the magnitude of influence inherent in these socialization domains is yet to be determined. Figure 15.3 summarizes some common themes inherent in the clinical clothing discussed in this chapter. Nurses must envision and decide what image best depicts their professional ideology and then incorporate this model into the organizational context.

Strategies for change must be developed within the two adult socialization institutions—nursing schools and clinical practice settings. Influ-

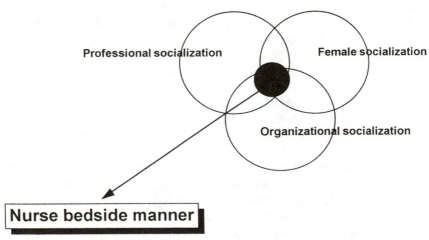

FIGURE 15.2. Socialization and bedside manner.

- **Colored smocks & uniforms**..occupation specific & servant status

- **Scrub suits**..function versus role specific

- **Military style uniform**..highlights status differentials

- **White dress uniform**..female stereotypes

- **Street clothes with white lab coat**..physicians & power

- **Street clothes**..role autonomy & no established stereotypes

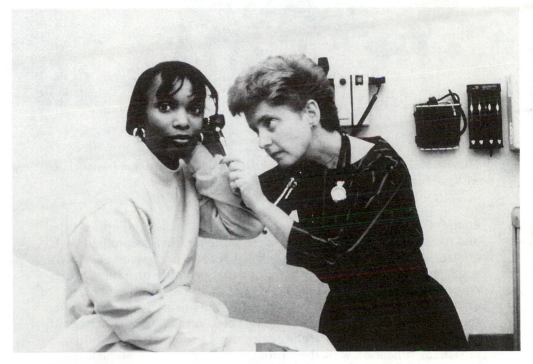

FIGURE 15.3. Clinical clothing as metaphor.
Nurses in street clothes deviate from expected stereotypical images and convey their professional status.

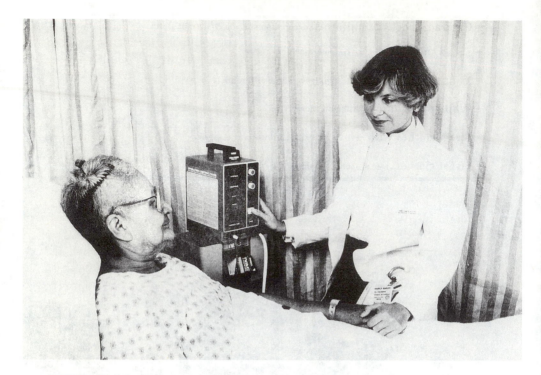

FIGURE 15.3 (cont.). Street clothing with a white laboratory coat is associated with physicians and power.

ences of female socialization on nursing practice must be appreciated and measured against persistent societal themes that perpetuate social control of women. Nursing leaders must recognize the elements in the social architecture of their institutions that promote or inhibit professional presentation of nurses, and consider these factors in relation to continuing historical themes prevalent in the hospital setting, such as the persistent undervaluing of nursing roles in relation to other health professionals. The social architecture must promote nurse status, increase identification with their professional group, and abolish media images of nurses as powerless, dependent sex objects, and assistants to physicians.

Nurse administrators can activate staff nurses to develop new communication patterns that disrupt sex role stereotypes, enhance nurses' self-esteem, build organizational trust, and model how professional nurses are to act (Barker, 1991; Bullough, 1992; Etzioni, 1964; Goffman, 1959; Gordon & Buresh, 1991). Basic to this mission is the provision of a safe work environment that fosters egalitarianism. Egalitarianism integrates co-workers into the organization and increases their maturity and autonomy. Interdisciplinary collegiality in institutions promotes productivity because this element meets both organizational and individual needs (Ouchi, 1982).

Social transformations must start at the top of organizational hierarchies. Nurse managers who recognize nursing care as equally important to other modalities will act to reinforce this ideology in all interdisciplinary arenas. The nurse administrator can use deliberative verbal and nonverbal communication strategies to strengthen organizational perceptions of nursing as a professional discipline. Careful attention to the social status implications of institutional communications during meetings, in memos, over loudspeakers, and with patients will support new metaphors of nursing within the work setting. Loudspeaker announcements—"Will Mary please come to the telephone?" reinforce the nonprofessional identity of staff. Childish name pins with only first names and telephone etiquette—"Hello, this is Mary"—also "advertise" subordinate nurse status. These naming nuances are even more poignant reminders of social hierarchy when combined with uniforms that reinforce, rather than refute, traditional nurse stereotypes.

Educators and leaders are in a position to promote and energize nurses by teaching strategies that foster deliberative communications that provide new metaphors for nursing—depictions of nurses as caring and competent professionals, equal in status to other health providers. This situation can create a social structure that increases nurses' self-worth, bedside image, and professional status in the workplace and community. Nursing leaders must first empower themselves by recognizing their caring role and contributions to quality nursing practice. The next step is striving to foster a common professional ideology among the nursing staff. Although this goal mandates addressing many organizational issues the promotion of more professional language and examination of the clinical dress metaphors inherent in various clinical settings, also contributes to this mission.

Nurse educators should introduce more theory about cultural influences and communications in the curriculum and reinforce these perspectives at the bedside. This situation is difficult when students practice in institutions where staff nurses model informal languaging and wear clothing devoid of professional, or sometimes even appropriate, design. Staff nurses convey powerful messages to nursing students about the role and status of the profession. A nursing professor role modeling formal address with patients feels like a salmon swimming upstream in institutions where staff reject these types of communications. Likewise, nursing professors must educate students at beginning practice levels about the importance of grooming and appropriate attire.

On an individual level, nurses must recognize how themes related to female socialization, societal stereotypes about women, and oppression permeate their own self-image. A clear understanding of these forces allows nurses to reclaim the social mandate that has always imbued nursing with great social value. It is the individual nurse at the bedside who provides the most powerful metaphor for patients. Attention to personal symbols of language and dress advance the actuality and image of the professional nurse. Those who respect themselves will convey this attitude to their colleagues and patients.

Nurses should also realize that their use of language and recognition of appearance can be used as tools to build self-esteem in others. Calling a teenager Ms. Smith and commenting on the appeal of clothing are excellent interventions to foster positive self-image. The patient recognizes the nurse's reinforcement of his or her adult status, which might promote more sense of responsibility for self-care. Nurses should also use this technique to build self-respect in their colleagues by taking care to use formal language when introducing colleagues to patients, groups, or families.

Central to the issue of social transformation in health care settings, is the question: Does naming and dressing really matter? Names and clothes continue to carry unconscious meanings and metaphors which convey messages to patients, families, other providers, and the public. Communicating contemporary professional images requires nurses to deviate from the expected stereotypic behavior. Individual nurses, administrators and educators must come together and recognize the need to shed traditional negative stereotypes about nurses that diminish our individual and collective images as competent professionals. Certainly, these stereotypes are reduced by excellent nursing care. However, deliberative communications strategies—both verbal and nonverbal—can accelerate professional recognition.

TOPICS FOR DISCUSSION

1. Are first or last names used for nurses in the hospital and health care settings you have worked in or visited? Are first or last names used for the other workers in these settings? Is the status hierarchy described by the authors apparent?
2. What are the historical implications of nursing uniforms?
3. What is your opinion regarding nursing uniforms?
4. Is image an important component of professionalism?

REFERENCES

Baggs, J. G., & Ryan, S. A. (1990). ICU nurse-physician collaboration and nursing satisfaction. *Nursing Economics, 8,* 386–392.

Baggs, J. C. & Schmitt, M. H. (1988). Collaboration between nurses and physicians. *Image, 20,* 145–149.

Barker, A. M. (1991). An emerging leadership paradigm. *Nursing and Health Care, 12,* 204–207.

Baszanger, I. (1985). Professional socialization and social control: From medical students to general practitioners. *Social Science and Medicine, 20,* 133–143.

Benner, P., & Wrubel, J. (1989). *The primacy of caring, stress and coping in health and illness.* Menlo Park, CA: Addison-Wesley.

Bennis, W., & Nanus, B. (1985). *Leaders: Strategies for taking charge.* New York: Harper and Row.

Bergren, M. D. (1992). *Shattering the stereotypes: Eulogy for the uniform,* Unpublished manuscript.

Blumhagen, D. W. (1979). The doctor's white coat: The image of the physician in modern America. *Annals of Internal Medicine, 91,* 111–116.

Brookfield, G., Douglas, A., Shapiro, R. S., & Clas, S. J. (1988). Some thoughts on being male in nursing. In J. Muff (Ed.), *Women's issues in nursing: Socialization, sexism, and stereotyping* (pp. 273–277). St. Louis: Mosby.

Bullough, B. (1992). Alternative models for specialty nursing practice. *Nursing and Health Care, 13,* 254–259.

Bullough, V. L. (1990). Nightingale, nursing and harassment. *Image, 2,* 4–7.

Campbell-Heider, N., & Pollock, D. (1987). Barriers to physician nurse collegiality: An anthropological perspective. *Social Science and Medicine, 25,* 421–425.

Davis, L. L. (1990). Social salience: What we notice first about a person. *Perceptual and Motor Skills, 71,* 334.

Diers, D. (1992). One liners. *Image, 24,* 75–77.

Etzioni, A. (1964). *Modern organizations.* Englewood Cliffs, NJ: Prentice-Hall.

Fagins, C., & Diers, D. (1983). Nursing as metaphor. *The New England Journal of Medicine, 309,* 116.

Flanagan, M. K. (1988). An analysis of nursing as a career choice. In J. Muff (Ed.), *Women's issues in nursing: Socialization, sexism, and stereotyping* (pp. 169–177). St. Louis: Mosby.

Forsythe, S. M., Drake, M. F., & Cox, C. A. (1984). Dress as an influence in the perceptions of management characteristics in women. *The Home Economics Research Journal, 13*(2), 112–121.

Goffman, E. (1959). *The presentation of self in everyday life.* Garden City, NJ: Doubleday.

Gordon, E., & Buresh, B. (1991, August 11). Nurses: They give care but get little in return. *Los Angeles Times.*

Hardin, S. B., & Benton, D. W. (1984). Fish or fowl: Nursing's ambivalence toward its symbols. *Journal of Nursing Education, 23,* 164–167.

Hedin, B. A. (1986). A case study of oppressed group behavior in nurses. *Image, 18,* 53–57.

Henley, N., & Freeman, J. (1988). The sexual politics of interpersonal behavior. In J. Muff (Ed.), *Women's issues in nursing: Socialization, sexism, and stereotyping* (pp. 83–94). Prospect Heights, IL: Waveland Press.

Joseph, N. (1986). *Uniforms and nonuniforms: Communication through clothing.* New York: Greenwood Press.

Kalisch, B. J., & Kalisch, P. A. (1985) Dressing for success. *American Journal of Nursing, 85*, 887–888, 890, 892–893.

Kalisch, P. A., & Kalisch, B. J. (1987). *The changing image of the nurse.* Menlo Park, CA: Addison-Wesley.

Kaiser, S. B. (1990). *The social psychology of clothing: Symbolic appearances in context.* New York: MacMillan.

Kaler, S. R., Levy, D. A., & Schall, M. (1989). Stereotypes of professional roles. *Image, 21*, 85–89.

Kearns, D. J. (1986). Do you know me? I'm a nurse. *RN, 49*, 63–64.

Little, D. (1984). The "strip tease" of nurse symbols or nurse dress code: No code. *Imprint, 31*, 49–52.

MacFarlane, M. E. (1990). The professional nurse: With or without a uniform. *Canadian Journal of Nursing Administration, 3*, 14–17.

Magnum, S., Garrison, C., Lind, C., Thackeray, R., & Wyatt, M. (1991). Perceptions of nurses' uniforms. *Image, 23*, 127–130.

Martin, M., Martin, J., & Sangster, E. (1986). Dress codes: Fashion statements that insult nurses. *Nursing, 16*, 33.

Miller, J. B., & Mothner, I. (1974). Psychological consequences of sexual inequality. *American Journal of Orthopsychiatry, 41*, 767–775.

Muff, J. (1988). *Women's issues in nursing: Socialization, sexism, and stereotyping.* Prospect Heights, IL: Waveland Press.

Ouchi, W. (1982). *Theory Z: How American business can meet the Japanese challenge.* New York: Avon.

Peplau, H. E. (1952). *Interpersonal relations in nursing.* New York: G.P. Putnam's Sons.

Peters, J., & Waterman, R. H. (1982). *In search of excellence.* New York: Harper & Row.

Raven, B. H. & Rubin, J. Z. (1976). *Social psychology.* New York: Wiley.

Reverby, S. (1987). A caring dilemma: Womanhood and nursing in historical perspective. *Nursing Research, 36*, 5–11.

Roberts, S. J. (1983). Oppressed group behavior: Implications for nursing. *Advances in Nursing Science, 5*, 21–30.

Rosenow, A. M. (1988). What is achievement in nursing? In J. Muff (Ed.), *Women's issues in nursing: Socialization, sexism, and stereotyping* (pp. 315–320). Prospect Heights, IL: Waveland Press.

'Safe uniform' debate. (1986). *American Journal of Nursing, 86*, 957–959.

Sampselle, C. (1990). The influence of feminist philosophy on nursing practice. *Image, 22*, 243–247.

Schutzenhofer, K. K. (1988). The problem of professional autonomy in nursing. *Health Care for Women International, 9*, 93–105.

Siegal, H. (1968). The nurse's uniform: Symbolic or sacrosanct. *Nursing Forum, 7*, 315–323.

Smoothy, V., Nightingale, C., & Harries, C. (1989). Should midwives wear uniforms? *Nursing Times, 85*, 38–40.

Sparrow, S. (1991). An exploration of the role of the nurses' uniform through a period of non-uniform wear on an acute medical ward. *Journal of Advanced Nursing, 16*, 116–122.

Stein, L. I., Watts, D. T., & Howell, T. (1990). Sounding board: The doctor-nurse game revisited. *The New England Journal of Medicine, 320*, 546–549.

Stephan, W. G. (1985). Intergroup relations. In G. Lindzey & E. Aronson (Eds.), *The handbook of social psychology* (pp. 599–658). New York: Random House.

Styles, M. M. (1982). *On nursing: Toward a new endowment.* St. Louis: Mosby.

Szasz, S. S. (1988). The tyranny of uniforms. In J. Muff (Ed.), *Women's issues in nursing: Socialization, sexism, and stereotyping* (pp. 397–401). Prospect Heights, IL: Waveland Press.

Vincenzi, A. E. (1991). Nurse Manner's guide to politically correct behavior. *Image, 23,* 193–194.

Zola, I. K. (1987). Structural constraints in the doctor–patient relationship: The case of non-compliance. In H. D. Schwartz (Ed.), *Dominant issues in medical sociology* (2nd ed) (pp. 203–209). New York: Random House.

Index